DISEASES OF SMALL DOMESTIC RODENTS

V.C.G. RICHARDSON *MA VetMB MRCVS*

SERIES EDITORS

J.B. SUTTON, JP, MRCVS

S.T. SWIFT, MA, VetMB, CertSAC

Blackwell Science

© 1997 by
Blackwell Science Ltd
Editorial Offices:
Osney Mead, Oxford OX2 0EL
25 John Street, London WC1N 2BL
23 Ainslie Place, Edinburgh EH3 6AJ
350 Main Street, Malden
  MA 02148 5018, USA
54 University Street, Carlton
  Victoria 3053, Australia
10, rue Casimir Delavigne
  75006 Paris, France

Other Editorial Offices:

Blackwell Wissenschafts-Verlag GmbH
Kurfürstendamm 57
10707 Berlin, Germany

Blackwell Science KK
MG Kodenmacho Building
7–10 Kodenmacho Nihombashi
Chuo-ku, Tokyo 104, Japan

First published 1997
Reprinted 2000

Set in 10/14 pt Souvenir
by DP Photosetting, Aylesbury, Bucks
Printed and bound in Great Britain by
MPG Books Ltd, Bodmin, Cornwall

The Blackwell Science logo is a trade mark
of Blackwell Science Ltd,
registered at the United Kingdom
Trade Marks Registry

DISTRIBUTORS

Marston Book Services Ltd
PO Box 269
Abingdon
Oxon OX14 4YN
(Orders: Tel: 01235 465500
        Fax: 01235 465555)

USA
Blackwell Science, Inc.
Commerce Place
350 Main Street
Malden, MA 02148 5018
(Orders: Tel: 800 759 6102
              781 388 8250
        Fax: 781 388 8255)

Canada
Login Brothers Book Company
324 Saulteaux Crescent
Winnipeg, Manitoba R3J 3T2
(Orders: Tel: 204 837 2987
        Fax: 204 837 3116)

Australia
Blackwell Science Pty Ltd
54 University Street
Carlton, Victoria 3053
(Orders: Tel: 03 9347 0300
        Fax: 03 9347 5001)

A catalogue record for this title
is available from the British Library
ISBN 0–632–04132–3

Library of Congress
Cataloging-in-Publication Data

Richardson, V.C.G.
    Diseases of small domestic rodents/
V.C.G. Richardson
    p.   cm. -(Library of veterinary
practice)
    Includes bibliographical references
(p.) and index.
    ISBN 0-632-04132-3
    1. Rodents-Diseases. 2.Rodents as
pets. I. Title. II. Series.
SF997.5.R64R53   1997
636.9'35-dc21   97-6214
                                 CIP

For further information on
Blackwell Science, visit our website:
www.blackwell-science.com

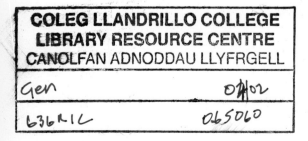

CONTENTS

RATS

PREFACE

Small rodents are becoming increasingly popular as pets, and as general practitioners we are called upon not only to treat their diseases, but also to advise on their health, husbandry and nutrition. Many of the diseases we encounter are the result of improper husbandry, so if we can advise on proper care and management of these pets we may be able to prevent at least a proportion of the conditions we see in practice. The aim of this book is to provide readily accessible and practical information about the upkeep of these species as pets, rather than as laboratory animals. It is hoped that it will be of help to veterinary surgeons in general practice, and to anyone who shares an interest in these smaller companion animals.

Each self-contained species section is divided into three chapters. Although this has necessitated some repetition, I feel it is more useful to keep each section species specific. In the 'Systems and Diseases' chapters drug treatments are referenced in brackets and, for each species, these treatments are detailed, providing dose rates and the components of proprietary preparations, which should enable alternatives to be found if necessary. Every effort has been made to ensure that all the dose rates are accurate; however, many drugs do not have specific licences for use in small rodents and dose rates given in the literature may have been extrapolated from larger mammals. Small rodents have higher metabolic rates and may metabolise drugs faster, thus requiring a higher dose rate and dosing frequency than larger mammals. Due care and sensible judgement must be taken when administering any drugs to rodents, remembering that, where possible, licensed products should be selected before non-licenced alternatives.

Throughout the book I have tried to include as much practical advice as possible, including remedies that have been tried and tested by hobbyists and pet keepers themselves (old-wives' remedies perhaps), because they have a definite place alongside modern medicine.

V.C.G. Richardson

CHINCHILLAS

There are two species of chinchilla, *Chinchilla lanigera* (with a long tail) and *Chinchilla brevicaudata* (with a short tail). It is *Chinchilla lanigera* which is commonly kept in captivity today.

Their natural environment is the Andes in South America where they are adapted to living on the snow-covered mountains, and the high valleys of Bolivia, Chile and Argentina. In 1923, 11 chinchillas were captured and bred in captivity, and it is from these animals that the majority of captive chinchillas are descended. Chinchillas were introduced as pets in the 1960s. They are hystricomorphic rodents and are mostly active from early evening into the night.

1 HUSBANDRY AND NUTRITION

Environment

In captivity, chinchillas do best at temperatures below 25°C (77°F) and 10–15°C (50–59°F) is ideal. Above 25°C they become distressed and susceptible to heat stroke, especially if the humidity is also high. If necessary, a dehumidifier should be used to keep the humidity at 70%. Chinchillas can survive at 0°C (32°F) providing they are free from damp and draughts, and at low temperatures they grow a very dense fur coat. Because of their susceptibility to heat stroke, their cages must not be placed in direct sunlight or close to radiators.

The room or building in which they are kept should be well ventilated and well lit. The atmosphere should not be too dry as this may predispose the animals to fur loss and respiratory disease. High humidity may also lead to infertility. The building should be positioned in the shade where possible. Painting the roof of the building with white or reflective aluminium paint will help keep the interior cooler in summer. Water can be sprayed over the roof on hot days.

Housing

Chinchillas are active gnawers and are best kept in wire mesh cages. They need plenty of space to exercise, and a cage of at least $2\,\text{m} \times 1\,\text{m} \times 0.45\,\text{m}$ (l × w × h) should be provided for a pair. To avoid limb injuries, the mesh should be no larger than $15\,\text{mm} \times 15\,\text{mm}$. Cages should be no higher than 45 cm because the chinchilla could fall, resulting in limb fractures or broken teeth. The floor should also be mesh, allowing urine and faeces to drop into a tray below. If a solid floor is used it increases the risk of faecal contamination and the spread of disease. It also increases the likelihood of fur staining.

3

A wooden nest box should be provided for each chinchilla, approximately 25 cm × 25 cm × 20 cm (l × w × h). Treated woods must be avoided as they may be toxic. A dust (sand) bath containing fine silver sand or silver sand and fuller's earth in a ratio of 9:1 should also be provided. Builder's sand will stain the coat and should not be used. The sand bath must be large enough for the chinchilla to roll over in. The sand helps to keep the fur clean by removing any dirt and grease, and helps satisfy the chinchilla's need to groom. The sand bath should not be left in the cage for more than 10–15 minutes as it may become soiled and contaminated. Prolonged sand-bathing may lead to dry skin if too many natural oils are stripped from the coat, and sand or dust in the air may increase the likelihood of conjunctivitis and respiratory disease. To maintain hygiene, the sand should be regularly sifted to remove any droppings. During the summer the sand bath should be used at the coolest time of day, because vigorous bathing in the heat may predispose animals to heatstroke.

The chinchilla likes to climb and should be provided with branches which can be safely gnawed, e.g. from apple or pear, or with wooden shelves. Pumice stones, pieces of walling blocks, e.g. Celcon, or hard bones should be provided for gnawing.

Stocking

Chinchillas can be kept singly, in pairs, in colonies or in polygamous units. In the last females are kept in single units and the male can travel between females via tunnels. The females are prevented from entering the tunnel by fitting them with a plastic collar which is just larger than the cage entrance. Pairs of females, or pairs of males will not live together, but a castrated male will live happily with a female if a non-breeding pair is required as pets.

Nutrition

Food should be provided in solid containers which cannot be spilled or soiled. Water can be provided by automatic drinkers or by drinker bottle. The spouts of drinkers must be stainless steel to prevent gnawing. Any build up of algae must be removed from the drinkers as it encourages the build up of *Pseudomonas aeruginosa* which will lead to diseases such as diarrhoea, oral ulceration and septicaemia.

In the wild, the chinchilla is a herbivore with a high fibre diet; most of the food that is available is nutritionally fairly poor. In captivity the diet is based on pellets, good quality hay which should be provided constantly from a hopper, rack or net to prevent soiling, and water. These foodstuffs are readily available and most closely approximate foods available in the wild. As a result of better nutrition, captive chinchillas are healthier and live longer than those in the wild.

Chinchillas should be fed regularly every day, generally in the early evening before their peak of activity, and again in the morning. Some chinchillas may develop convulsions if fed long after their preferred feeding time and, if fed late, they may become fur chewers.

Nutritional requirements

- Protein: 15% (to increase during pregnancy and lactation)
- Carbohydrate: 35%
- Fat: 4%
- Fibre: 30%
- Minerals: 6%
- Moisture and trace elements: 10%

Most pellets contain an average of 18.5% protein, 3.5% oil, 7.5% fibre, 7.5% ash (minerals) and vitamins A, D and E. Pellets should be fed fresh as their vitamin content decreases with age. An average adult will eat 20 g pellets a day. Where possible, pellets specially formulated for chinchillas should be fed, but if these are unavailable rabbit or guinea pig pellets can be used.

Because pellets do not contain sufficient fibre, the deficit is made up by good hay. However, the quality of hay and its nutritional value may be variable. Clover and lucerne hays are the best, but the least available. The calcium content of hay varies from 1.5% in good clover hay to 0.3% in poorer hays, while the protein content can vary from 16% in good clover hay to 6% in timothy hays. On average, alfalfa contains 14% protein and is sold as compressed hay cubes or blocks which are an ideal source of fibre and useful for gnawing. Hay must be stored dry because damp hay may become mouldy, causing the production of fatal toxins. Hay that is too coarse should not be fed as it may cause impaction, intussusception or rectal prolapse. Poor or damp hay will also cause diarrhoea.

A low protein diet will result in unthriftiness and dry, weak fur. Fur chewing may also occur. Poor nutrition causes increased mortality in young, decreased milk production in lactating females, and poorer performance (i.e. poor condition, reduced fertility) in adults. However, if chinchillas are fed diets that are too high in protein (greater than 28%) the normal hair fibres become weak and wavy, giving a cotton-like appearance. This condition is known as 'cotton fur'.

Unsaturated fatty acids: Chinchillas require unsaturated fatty acids to maintain fur growth and quality, and for a healthy skin. Diets deficient in linoleic and arachidonic acids lead to cutaneous ulcers and reduced hair growth (occasionally mistakenly referred to as fungus or fur slip). Chinchillas cannot make these unsaturated fatty acids and so must obtain adequate amounts from their diet.

Vitamin A: Vitamin A is required for the maintenance of healthy eyes, skin, coat and the reproductive system. Deficiency can lead to watery eyes, dull fur, fetal resorption or abortion, or the birth of weak, blind litters. Many chinchillas are unable to manufacture vitamin A from its precursor carotene and so may require dietary supplements. Food pellets usually contain sufficient amounts of the vitamin, but it can also be given in a vegetable oil base (along with the other fat soluble vitamins D and E). Cod-liver oil should not be used as it quickly turns rancid and the vitamins are destroyed. Similarly, old pellets should not be used because the vitamin content decreases with time. During pregnancy and lactation, or if an animal is showing signs of deficiency, large doses of vitamin A can be given (up to 2000 i.u. daily).

Carotene can build up in the tissues of the chinchilla, where it causes a condition known as 'yellow ears'. Discoloration of the fat and ears occurs, followed by the abdomen and perineal region. This is caused by a deficiency in vitamin E, choline (a member of the vitamin B complex) of the amino acid methionine, which act together to facilitate the breakdown of carotene. However, the condition improves when the three are supplemented in the diet.

Vitamin D, calcium and phosphorus: Vitamin D, calcium and phosphorus are important for the proper calcification of bones and teeth: vitamin D is formed when the skin is exposed to sunlight, and it is also added to pellet feed.

Calcium and phosphorus are required in a ratio of between 1:1 and 2:1. An imbalance will produce musculoskeletal weakness and cramping, especially in pregnant or young, growing chinchillas. One of the best sources of calcium and phosphorus is sterilised bone meal or bone flour, because it provides calcium and phosphorus in the correct ratio, containing 30% Ca and 15% P. This can be given at a maintenance rate of half a teaspoonful twice a week.

The nutritional requirements for calcium are variable depending upon the state of the animal. The requirement increases twofold during lactation, and even more if the female is carrying another litter at the same time as the result of a post-partum mating.

Nutritional requirements (Ca)	Growth	Maintenance	Pregnancy	Lactation
% of dry matter kg	0.4%	0.3%	0.4%	0.6%

The diet of nursing females can be supplemented with evaporated milk diluted 1:1 with boiled water, or with skimmed milk at a rate of 2 table-spoonsful (30 ml) at 10 days before parturition into the lactation period. Skimmed milk is preferable as it is lower in calories but still contains calcium and vitamins. Cows' milk contains too much fat.

Nursing females can exhibit a condition similar to milk fever in cattle, which is associated with hypocalcaemia. It occurs typically 2–3 weeks post-partum. Clinical signs are hind limb paralysis, gastrointestinal stasis and bloat. These signs can be reduced by a slow intraperitoneal injection of 100 mg/kg calcium gluconate. The condition, known as tympanites, may be prevented by suitable dietary supplementation.

Titbits

Chinchillas are susceptible to diet induced diarrhoea, which can be caused by the introduction of too many extra food treats. Raisins are popular, but no more than two should be given daily. Alternative supplements are small pieces of apple ($\frac{1}{6}$ apple once a week), $\frac{1}{6}$ carrot, small quantities of dandelion, and shepherd's purse. Dried fruits can be given in small quantities but dried coconut should be avoided because it swells inside the stomach as it rehydrates. Nuts and sunflower seeds should not be used because of their high fat content, and fruits that have stones, such as plums and cherries, should also be avoided because the stones may be toxic.

2 SYSTEMS AND DISEASES

THE SKIN

It is the nature of the dense fur coat that was responsible for the original popularity of the chinchilla. The thick coat makes the chinchilla less susceptible to external parasites than other rodents. To maintain a healthy coat it is important to provide a dust/sand bath for 10–15 minutes daily. By rolling in the sand the chinchilla is able to keep the coat clean and remove any excess grease. A greasy, matted coat is most likely if the humidity of the air is high. The sand bath can also be a useful vehicle for topical skin preparations.

In the wild, the chinchilla is accustomed to low environmental temperatures which stimulate hair growth to form a dense coat. In captivity, the optimum temperature is 15–20°C (59–68°F). A dry atmosphere, such as that in a centrally heated room, may cause heavy hair loss.

Ringworm

The commonest cause is *Trichophyton mentagrophytes*; *Microsporum canis* and *Microsporum gypseum* have also been isolated.

Clinical signs: There is hair loss on extremities, ears, nose and feet. The lesions may be hyperaemic and crusty.

Treatment: Oral griseofulvin at a dose of 25 mg/kg twice daily or 50 mg/kg daily for at least a month should be given. Grisovin tablets (Tx 6) contain 125 mg griseofulvin and an eighth of a tablet can be given twice daily to an adult, or one quarter of a tablet daily. Care should be taken with pregnant animals as griseofulvin may be teratogenic. Lime sulphur dips are useful, and antifungal powders can be added to the dust bath to prevent

8

spread of the condition. Human athlete's foot powder containing tolnaftate 1% w/w can be used for this purpose, and a tablespoonful (15 g) of this powder can be added to the sand bath. As a preventative measure tolnaftate can be mixed in with the sand bath on a monthly basis.

Ectoparasites

Due to the dense nature of the fur coat external parasites are extremely rare. Fleas may be caught from an in-contact dog or cat. The safest ectoparasiticide spray is one containing pyrethrin (Tx 12). Flowers of sulphur can also be used as a dusting powder.

Dietary deficiencies

Cotton fur

Clinical signs: The hair fibres are weak and wavy, giving a cotton-like appearance. This occurs if the pellet ration is too high in protein. The average diet should only contain 15–18% protein. If chinchilla pellets are unavailable, rabbit or guinea pig ones should be used. Rations for poultry are unsuitable as they are too high in protein.

Vitamin A deficiency

Please see page 6.

Vitamin E deficiency

Chinchillas require vitamin E, along with methionine and choline, to convert carotene into vitamin A in the liver. If carotene builds up it causes a yellow discolouration of the ears (yellow ears) which may progress to discolouration of the ventral abdomen. The chinchilla may also develop small well-circumscribed swellings on the ventral abdomen (similar to vitamin E-responsive dermatitis in dogs). The condition should respond to dietary supplementation with choline, methionine and vitamin E.

Unsaturated fatty acid deficiency

A deficiency of linoleic, linolenic and arachidonic acids will cause reduced hair growth, poor hair coats and cutaneous ulcers. Symptoms range from a degree of dry, flaky skin to larger areas of hair loss, which are occasionally pruritic. This condition is sometimes referred to as fungus.

The condition will improve with supplementation, and 5–10 mg/day evening primrose oil can be given. If the skin is sore a cream containing linoleic acid can be applied.

Zinc deficiency

This will also cause a dull, poor coat. Affected individuals will be in poor condition and have areas of patchy hair loss.

Fur slip

Chinchillas are able to shed their hair readily if roughly handled, or during fighting. The hair is lost leaving a patch of bare skin, with no inflammation. Chinchillas that are susceptible to stress may lose their fur more readily, and hair regrowth may take as long as 4–6 months.

Fur chewing

Clinical signs: Fur chewing is seen either as the result of barbering by other chinchillas, or from self-mutilation. Affected chinchillas are generally nervous and susceptible to stress. Hair loss is generally seen over the shoulders and sides of the body, and the fur has a moth-eaten, chewed appearance. Often the darker undercoat remains, and has a poor, dry appearance; it may be associated with dandruff. The paws may also be chewed.

Causes: The aetiology of fur chewing is not fully understood, and there are many different factors involved, including the following.

- *Heredity.* It is thought that there may be a familial tendency towards hair-chewing. It may be that some lines are more stressed and nervous, and therefore more likely to chew. Severely affected individuals are best not bred from.
- *Environment.* Boredom, overcrowding, small cages and aggression may all cause fur chewing. Cages that are kept in draughts predispose to the problem, as does a high environmental temperature. At higher temperatures, chinchillas moult more readily and are more likely to be stressed. They may also chew themselves in an attempt to keep cool.

- *Diet*. Chinchillas on a balanced diet with a healthy coat are least likely to chew. If the diet is deficient in vitamins or unsaturated fatty acids the fur will be poorer, and chewing more likely. A monotonous diet may lead to boredom and increased chewing. A diet that includes plenty of roughage (e.g. good hay) and a small amount of green food may prevent fur chewing. Some dietary variation, without causing digestive upset, may also prevent the condition.
- *Concurrent illness*. Any factors which reduce the general health of the chinchilla will predispose to fur chewing. Individuals with liver, kidney or digestive dysfunction may all fur chew, and these conditions should be attended to. Where poor digestion is the problem this may be improved by the use of a probiotic (e.g.Tx 5. Avipro).
- *Behaviour*. Some sources suggest that fur chewing is a vice.

Prevention: The environmental surroundings may need to be adjusted. Chinchillas thrive if the temperature is lowered, providing they are protected from draughts. Cage sizes must be generous, and if necessary extra nest boxes, low shelves, branches and pumice stones added to relieve boredom. Roughage (hay) should be constantly available. The diet should be supplemented with adequate vitamins and unsaturated fatty acids and bone meal.

Treatment: The affected individual will not regrow any fur whilst the short dark undercoat is present. The dark dead fur must be plucked from the affected areas, and a soothing cream (e.g. Tx 14. Dermisol) applied onto the pale skin. As the condition improves the skin will change from pink to a dark blue colour. It may be necessary to use an Elizabethan collar to prevent further self-mutilation in the short term.

Fur rings

Clinical signs: Fur rings occur at mating when fur becomes wrapped around the male's penis, often causing paraphimosis. This ring will act as a constricting band around the penis resulting in pain, difficulty urinating, and damage of the entrapped organ. The chinchilla will attempt to groom the ring free, but in some cases is unable to, leading to excessive grooming.

Occasionally smaller rings are formed which can be drawn into the foreskin, and are less immediately obvious. Males should always be examined after mating.

Treatment: The penis should be gently lubricated with petroleum jelly e.g. Vaseline. The fur ring should be carefully teased open and cut off gently with scissors.

Endocrinopathies

Alopecia may be associated with abnormalities of the adrenal or thyroid gland. Chinchillas that fur chew often have hyperactive adrenal and thyroid glands, although it is unknown whether these cause the alopecia, or have become overactive in order to stimulate new hair growth once the fur has been chewed.

Abscesses

These form as a result of bite wounds or traumatic injury. The causal bacteria are usually *Staphylococcus* and *Streptococcus* spp.

Treatment: The abscess can be lanced and flushed with an antiseptic solution or a dilute solution of hydrogen peroxide, and packed with anti-biotic. Alternatively the abscess can be surgically removed. In either instance antibiotics should be given by injection or orally (Tx 1–4).

Minor wounds

These occur due to traumatic injury or from minor fights, often between kits when competing for milk.

Small wounds can be bathed with saline, or mild antiseptic solution, and an antiseptic wound powder applied. Ster-zac powder (Tx 15) is available from pharmacies and contains 0.33% hexachlorophane, 3% zinc oxide and sterilised talc, and is effective in preventing staphylococcal infections. Veterinary wound powders are also suitable.

Cysts

Clinical signs: Discreet soft tissue swellings in the skin.

Treatment: Cysts can either be removed surgically under a general anaesthetic, or can be drained by needle aspiration.

THE REPRODUCTIVE SYSTEM

The chinchilla is a hystricomorphic rodent and, like the guinea pig, has a long gestation period resulting in young which are born at an advanced stage of development, fully furred and with their eyes open.

- Litter size: 1–5 (average 2)
- Birth weight: 30–60 g
- Weaning age: 6–8 weeks
- Puberty: 4–8 months
- Age to start breeding: 8 months
- Breeding life: 10 years
- Oestrus cycle: 24–45 days
- Post-partum oestrus: fertile (40%)
- Gestation: 111 days

Sexing

In the male, the anogenital distance is much larger than the female. The female has a slit-like vulva which is generally closed, apart from 3–5 days around each season. The urethral orifice is at the end of a genital papilla which protrudes from the vulva (Figure 2.1).

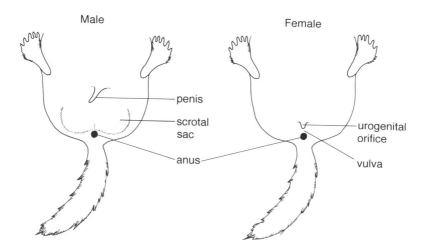

Figure 2.1 External genitalia.

Breeding

Chinchillas are seasonally polyoestrous, and in the northern hemisphere most matings take place in late autumn, with litters beginning to arrive in early spring (March). If the female remates after parturition a second litter is born in the summer.

Pairing

Chinchillas can be bred from at 7 months of age and onwards. They can be bred as pairs, or in a polygamous unit, where one male may have access to several females. When introducing a pair together for the first time it should be done slowly. Initially they can be placed in two wire cages side by side, or the female introduced in a small wire cage put inside the male's cage so that they can scent each other; the final pairing can be done by placing them together in a neutral cage. Pairing is best done during the day when they are least active. Young animals may form a pair quite quickly, whilst older animals may take several days to accept each other.

Mating

Various signs may indicate that the pair are ready to breed. The male may make a cooing, chuckling noise and both sexes may rub their chins on the floor or nest box. The female's vagina will become opened and reddened; the female's nipples may also be reddened. At the beginning of oestrus the female may eject a small wax plug (the oestrus plug). After mating, which generally takes place at night, the female produces another plug, the copulatory plug or stopper. These stoppers are a mixture of female and male reproductive fluids and remain in the female's vagina for a few hours after mating to prevent the loss of semen. These plugs are then shed, and are a good indication that mating has taken place. The stoppers can be 3 cm long; initially they are white and full of mucus, but shrivel up and change to a yellow colour when exposed to air. A stopper is less common if the mating is at the post-partum oestrus. After mating the male should be checked for the presence of a fur ring (see Skin section) and if necessary this should be removed.

The pair can be kept together during gestation and parturition. However, approximately 12 hours after parturition the female will exhibit a post-partum oestrus which lasts for 2 days. This oestrus is fertile; mating should only be allowed if the female is in good physical condition and is only caring for a small litter. Females should not have more than two litters in succession before having a rest. The male should not be kept with the first litter after their weaning age, but visual contact can be maintained by keeping him in an adjacent cage.

Gestation

Gestation lasts on average 111 days. By day 90 the female should have abdominal enlargement, and her nipples will be reddened. Pregnancy can be confirmed by radiographic examination if necessary. Experienced breeders may be able to palpate the fetuses from 60 days of pregnancy. Monitoring weight gain is a safer way of detecting pregnancy; a weight gain of 25–30 g/month is expected initially, increasing in the last month of gestation.

In the last 4 weeks of pregnancy the female should receive a balanced diet to ensure adequate vitamin intake. Brassicas (kale, cabbage) should be avoided because they cause bloat at this time. Chinchillas do not build nests; however, the provision of a nest box is useful to encourage a place for littering, otherwise the young will be born on the cage floor. Young that are born on the cage floor are more susceptible to hypothermia; the cage should be free from draughts, and if necessary a heating pad should be provided if the external temperature is low.

Complications during pregnancy

Abortions

The premature loss of young can occur at any stage of gestation. This may be the result of poor nutrition, a concurrent illness, stress (even loud noises may startle a pregnant female) and trauma such as a fall. Unskilful palpation may also cause miscarriage or abortion.

Clinical signs: Aborted fetuses may be present in the cage; however, the female often eats them. The female may have a bloody vaginal discharge, or a foul smelling serous discharge. Weight loss in a female previously assumed pregnant may also indicate that she has aborted. Occasionally all that is seen is a wetting of the nose and forepaws of the female which then dries off.

Treatment: Radiographic examination can be used to confirm whether all, or part of the litter have been lost. If the uterus is empty it can be flushed with a saline solutioin, and an oxytetracycline or neomycin preparation instilled. Systemic antibiosis may also be necessary (Tx 1–4).

Parturition

A few days before the anticipated parturition date, the sand bath should be removed to avoid particles entering the vagina and causing infection. Before the onset of parturition the female may become aggressive towards the male; she may also refuse food. Parturition generally takes place in the early morning; it is generally a quick process, often of only a few minutes duration, and the maximum length is 4 hours. Parturition commences with the loss of amniotic fluid, and the genitals, mouth and nose of the female will appear wet at this time. The delivery of the young should follow soon after. The female will deliver the young from her vagina by pulling with her mouth, and if the birth is difficult or the young get stuck in the birth canal she may be seen to cannibalise them. The young are precocious; they are born fully furred and with their eyes open. The female will eat all the placentas (afterbirths).

Following parturition the vagina may remain open for 3–4 days, and sand baths should not be given at this time to minimise the risks of metritis.

Problems during or after parturition

Dystocia

Dystocia is rare but will occur if there is fetal malpresentation, an oversized youngster, or uterine inertia. Inertia may occur if the female is in poor condition and undernourished. Occasionally two fetuses may be present in the birth canal simultaneously, resulting in difficulties during parturition.

Clinical signs: Affected females may have a wet nose from the initial loss of amniotic fluid, which then dries without subsequent birth of a litter, a bloody vaginal discharge, or be distressed and lick and tug at their vulva.

Treatment: With rapid intervention Caesarean section is rewarding, and the young are generally very active as soon as they are delivered. Caesarean sections carried out after dystocia has been evident for many hours are less likely to produce viable young.

Uterine inertia can initially be treated with an intramuscular injection of

1 i.u. oxytocin. Oral calcium in the form of Collo-Cal D (Tx 24) can be given at a dose of 0.5 ml/kg. If this does not induce parturition within 4 hours, Caesarean section should be considered.

Occasionally after littering there may be a stillborn or mummified fetus left in the uterus. The female may appear restless and ignore the newborns. The presence of such a fetus can usually be determined by radiography, and its expulsion can be encouraged by an intramuscular injection of 1 i.u. oxytocin. If this is unsuccessful the fetus must be removed by Caesarean section.

Caesarean section

The sooner that dystocia is recognised and Caesarean section carried out, the better the chances of survival of the female and her kits. If, however, the female is already tired or in poor condition the outcome may be less favourable, because the female is less likely to survive the anaesthetic and surgery. The kits are born at an advanced state of development, and are often very lively soon after delivery.

Surgical procedure: For details of anaesthesia and surgical pre-paration see Chapter 3. The chinchilla is placed in dorsal recumbency and the surgery carried out through a midline incision. The uterus should be opened close to its bifurcation, and the young and placentas delivered through this incision. The wound should then be closed using an inverting continuous suture of catgut or other absorbable thread. Closure of the peritoneum and muscle can be done as one layer, preferably using an interrupted suture pattern. The skin can then be closed using a subcuticular continuous absorbable suture, e.g. Vicryl, which avoids the stress of suture removal at a later date and produces a neat wound which does not interfere with the suckling of the young.

Post-operative care: Post-operatively the female should be given an intramuscular injection of 1 i.u. oxytocin, and 5–10 ml subcutaneous fluid replacement. It may be necessary to supplement the diet of the young whilst the female is recovering, as it may take 2–3 days for her milk supply to become adequate.

Metritis and pyometritis

The acute form of metritis occurs shortly after parturition; it may be caused by a retained placenta or fetus, a dirty environment, or follow damage to the birth canal resulting from a difficult birth, or intervention with unsterile instruments at the time of birth. Chronic metritis may occur later as a result of a retained or mummified fetus.

Pyometritis may occur in females that have never been bred from.

Clinical signs: The chinchilla has a purulent vaginal discharge, is anorexic and pyrexic. The vulva becomes swollen and reddened and the female may develop agalactia, resulting in restless, hungry kits. The female may exhibit abdominal contractions, and have a stiff hind-limb gait.

Treatment: Cases of acute metritis may be unresponsive to treatment. The uterus should be flushed with an antiseptic (such as a saline solution), and antibiotics can be introduced per vagina. An older remedy is to flush the uterus with 25 ml of warm water to which 3 drops of vinegar have been added. Systemic antibiotics should also be given (Tx 1–4). An injection of oxytocin will help any debris from the womb to be expelled. Any young kits will need to be fostered or hand reared if they are to survive.

In cases of chronic metritis and pyometritis an ovariohysterectomy should be performed. The uterus is often inflamed and dark red to purple in colour when it is removed. Systemic antibiotics should also be given (Tx 1–4).

Puerperal septicaemia

This condition may be a sequel to metritis or pyometritis if the bacteria or their endotoxins gain entry to the blood stream and cause septicaemia.

Clinical signs: A uterine discharge is seen, accompanied by agalactia, depression, anorexia and collapse. Symptoms usually develop within 12–24 hours of parturition. In the early stages the chinchilla may have a temperature of 40–41°C (104–105°F).

Treatment: This is rarely successful in severe cases. Antibiotics should be given, by subcutaneous or intraperitoneal injection. An anti-inflammatory drug, (e.g. flunixin Tx 17. Finadyne) can be given to combat endotoxic shock. Warmth, fluids and supportive nursing are required. As for metritis the uterus can be flushed.

It is usually necessary to foster or hand rear the youngsters.

Agalactia

The female usually comes into full milk production 3 days after parturition. Signs that the young are suckling are that they are full-bellied and contented, whilst the mother is damp around the nipples.

If there is little or no milk available for the young they will become aggressive, restless, cry and adopt a hunched tucked-up appearance. The female may also become aggressive towards the youngsters as they constantly pester her for food, often seriously injuring them. The young may bite each other on the nose in their attempts to fight for milk.

The female should be examined after parturition and her milk supply checked. If the teats are difficult to find amongst the fur it is useful to clip the fur away from both sets of nipples to make them more readily accessible. With large litters it may be necessary to supplement their diet in the early stages, or foster some to a female with a smaller litter. The young are born with food reserves sufficient to last them for the first 12 hours during which they do not need to suckle; a female that has little milk at parturition may come into milk at this time. Youngsters should at first be left with their mother because their presence will stimulate her milk flow, but if after 12 hours the female still has little milk, supplementation of the diet of the young or fostering some of the litter should be considered.

Treatment: If necessary, milk production can be stimulated with an intramuscular injection of 1 i.u. oxytocin. If agalactia is only a problem in the first 3 days whilst the milk production is developing, the young can be hand fed at this stage. If agalactia is a symptom of another condition such as metritis then this must be treated too, and the young fostered if necessary. Females with large litters should receive good rations of chinchilla pellets, on which milk powder or Bemax can be sprinkled to support them during lactation.

Damaged teats

If the female has a poor milk supply or a large litter, the young may bite the teats (they are born with their incisor teeth) in their urgency to feed. The female will become irritable towards the litter and in some cases injure them fatally.

Females should be examined regularly, and damaged teats treated with antiseptic bathing and an antibiotic cream, or Kamillosan cream (Tx 13) (a herbal preparation which is safe if ingested by the young). If the teats are very sore the young should be hand reared or fostered.

Caked milk glands

Clinical signs: Sometimes teats may become caked with excess milk, which dries and makes the teat inaccessible. This may occur if the female produces more milk than her young can drain off, or if she develops her milk supply prematurely before the young are born. The females should be checked for caked glands while they are susceptible, from 1 week before parturition through to the first 3 weeks of lactation. The teat may then become congested and develop mastitis.

Treatment: The teats should be bathed and, if necessary, the fur clipped from around them and any excess of milk stripped from them. In the case of mastitis the glands must be bathed regularly, warm poultices can be applied for up to 20 minutes two or three times daily, and antibiotics given orally or by injection (Tx 1–4).

Petroleum jelly, e.g. Vaseline, can be put on a sore teat to prevent the young sucking from it and causing the female pain. Alternatively, a herbal preparation (Tx 13. Kamillosan) can be applied to the nipples two or three times daily to aid healing. This preparation is safe for the suckling young.

Cannibalism

This may occur if the female is nervous, or is disturbed excessively after parturition. A female that is over enthusiastic when chewing the afterbirths and umbilical cords may inadvertently damage her young.

Lack of water at a time when the female has increased thirst may result in cannibalism. The female is also likely to attack her young if she has little milk and they persistently worry her. Some females may have a genetic tendency towards cannibalism, and these should not be used for breeding.

Occasionally the young are damaged by trampling, especially if the male is left with the female to breed again. This may be prevented by providing a shelf under which the young can escape, or by removing the male.

Tympanites

Clinical signs: In females bloat associated with gastric stasis is observed, usually 2–3 weeks post-partum. The hind legs may also become paralysed. Tympanites is thought to be associated with hypocalcaemia.

Treatment: Affected chichillas may respond to an intraperitoneal injection of calcium gluconate, at a dose of 94–140 mg/kg.

Lactating females that may be at risk (those in poor condition or with large litters) can be given calcium supplementation; powdered milk can be sprinkled on their food or they can be given oral calcium and vitamin D (Tx 24. Collo-Cal D) at a dose of 0.5 ml/kg daily in the early stages of lactation.

Constipation

Female chinchillas may become constipated at any time during the first week post-partum. The droppings become small, scant and dry, and the milk supply may dry up. Raisins can be given as a laxative, or even as a precautionary measure after parturition. Alternatively the female can be given up to 2 ml syrup of figs daily until the condition resolves.

Revival of young

One of the commonest causes of loss of young is hypothermia, if they are born out of the nest box or stray away from the warmth of the female. A chilled youngster can be gently held in warm water, submerged to the neck, and then towelled vigorously to increase its body temperature. The chest can be gently massaged and squeezed. A heat pad or the warmth of an airing cupboard will then help maintain its temperature; the ideal environmental temperature is 27°C (80°F).

Any weak young are best isolated, warmed and hand fed. If kept with the litter they are likely to be pushed out by the stronger offspring and chilled.

Problems with the male

Swollen penis

Swelling of the penis may be caused by a fur ring which must be removed with care. Urolithiasis, or infection secondary to trauma may be other causes requiring appropriate treatment.

Clinical signs: The penis is flaccid, but swollen and inflamed with the foreskin retracted. If it remains in this condition for long it may become blue and necrotic because the blood circulation is disrupted.

Swollen testicles

In a male that is ready for breeding, or in a male that has just mated, the testicles may be enlarged and swollen. Unless the testicles are hard and painful this is generally quite normal.

Castration

Chinchillas have inguinal canals which are open from birth, and it is important to close them to prevent herniation of the abdominal contents after surgery. The chinchilla is able to completely withdraw its testicles into the abdomen, but gentle pressure on the caudal abdomen should return them to the scrotum.

Surgical procedure: A bilateral scrotal incision is made, and castration is generally done by the open technique. The tunic is incised, exposing the testicle and the spermatic cord. The vas deferens and the spermatic cord are ligated, as is the testicular ligament. The tunic is then closed, and this is followed by closure of the inguinal canal. The skin is generally closed with simple interrupted sutures of an absorbable material, e.g. Vicryl, to avoid the stress of suture removal.

Orphans

Fostering

If possible the foster mother should have a litter of approximately the same age as the orphans. However, if she already has a litter of two or three she may not be able to accept further kits.

If the orphan is to be accepted it is best to put a dab of mentholated ointment, e.g. Vick, on its back, and the foster mother's kits should also have some, so that all the young smell the same, and the orphan is less likely to be rejected. The litter must be watched closely to ensure that the orphan is accepted.

If no chinchilla mother is available a nursing female guinea pig would make a suitable alternative. Also suitable would be a chinchilla with an older litter ready for weaning, because the young kits can be weaned and the orphans introduced after a few hours.

Hand rearing

If a foster mother is not available the kits can be hand reared. Hand rearing may also be necessary if a female has a large litter, or if a foster mother has a large extended family. Because the young are born at an advanced stage of development, they take readily to hand rearing. It is useful for the kits to have some adult companion (perhaps their father or a female guinea pig) to provide warmth and company. Even if the adult animal does not take part in the feeding process it may often become involved with the cleaning and grooming of the young.

The young are born with enough reserves to last them for 12 hours before they need to be fed, unless they are very undersized in which instance feeding should commence straight away. The orphans can be fed on evaporated milk diluted 1:1 with boiled water, and fed through an eye dropper. The baby should be held in an upright position so that it can swallow easily. Care must be taken not to force milk into the mouth because this may cause a fatal inhalation pneumonia. If the young get bloated on this mixture it must be made more dilute (30% evaporated milk, 60% boiled water and 10% glucose).

Initially the young will need to be fed every 2 hours. If no adult is available to clean the young, after feeding the orphan must be massaged over the lower abdomen and genitals with warm, damp cotton wool to stimulate it to urinate and defaecate. After the first week the milk mixture can be thickened with a little baby cereal (e.g. Milupa baby rice). A drop of multivitamins (1 drop per baby per day) can be added and also a probiotic (e.g. Tx 5. Avipro) to maintain a healthy gut flora.

Feeding on a less regular basis of three or four times a day may be required until the young are at least 45 days old, and sometimes up to 60 days. It is useful to keep a regular check on the kits' weight, especially after hand feeding has stopped; if they fail to gain weight, they may require further feeding. The kits will start to eat solid food 10 days after parturition, but they still require milk to help them digest their food properly.

Infertility

The female

- *Poor management.* Females that are in poor condition, undernourished, or that have had several sequential litters may fail to breed. These females should be fed properly to improve their body condition before being mated. Extra protein in the form of milk powder, multi-vitamins, and wheatgerm or wheatgerm oil (as a source of vitamin E) can be given to improve condition and fertility. Underfeeding and over-breeding will also affect the fertility of the male (see below).

Breeding is 'contagious' in a unit. The sights, sound and scent of a breeding pair may well stimulate breeding activity in neighbouring pairs. With a pair that are reluctant to breed, it may be beneficial to move them closer to a sexually active pair.

- *Obesity*. This is less common, but an overweight female will become lazy and reluctant to breed. The diet should be corrected, and adequate provision given for exercise. Fattening treats should be avoided, because most individuals will eat these first in preference to their regular ration.
- *Age*. A healthy female may have a breeding life span of up to 10 years. However, as the female becomes older the interval between her litters may become longer, and her litter size smaller. Young females that are born late in the season may not breed until they are 18 months of age. This is because they are not sexually mature enough to breed in the breeding season of their birth, but breed during the subsequent season.
- *Infection*. The presence of concurrent infection, e.g. metritis, or adhesions in the uterine tubes as a result of previous infection may result in sterility. Flushing the uterus with an antibiotic/antiseptic solution may make further breeding possible.
- *Mummified fetuses*. Fetuses that are lost during gestation are generally resorbed or aborted. However, occasionally they will become mummified and remain in the uterus and hinder further pregnancies. They are found in females that have previously bred, and also in females that have been with a male but never bred. Mummified fetuses can be identified by palpation, and depending on the fetal age at mummification, by radiography.

The male

- *Obesity*. Overweight males become lazy and are reluctant to breed. Their diet must be corrected and they should be given adequate opportunity to exercise.
- *Inexperience*. A young male, especially if it is submissive, may appear infertile. The temperament of the chinchillas must be considered when pairing the breeding stock. The male should be examined; if his testicles are small or undescended he is unlikely to be ready for breeding.

- *Overuse.* If a male is mated too frequently, or used in a polygamous breeding system he may become sterile. He must be rested and fed well before rebreeding. A vitamin E supplement (wheatgerm or wheatgerm oil) may be useful.

THE URINARY SYSTEM

The kidneys

Changes in kidney pathology may only be noticed at post-mortem examination; clinical signs may not be evident in the living animal. Primary kidney problems are rare; the changes in the kidney are usually secondary to another disease process. Certain drugs, or mouldy foods may lead to kidney damage. Chinchillas that are kept in a cold and damp environment have a predisposition to kidney disease.

Acute nephritis

Clinical signs: These include anorexia, constipation later followed by diarrhoea, and pyrexia. The chinchilla may have a stiff gait and exhibit pain over the kidneys. The condition carries a poor prognosis.

Treatment: Supportive nursing, warmth and fluids are needed. Oral fluid replacement is preferred, and glucose water should be given little and often. Orange juice can be added to the glucose water to increase its palatability.

Chronic nephritis

Clinical signs: There is loss of appetite and weight loss. Haematuria may be present. Often the kidney damage is advanced before clinical signs are evident. A chronic purulent nephritis may follow an abortion or metritis, and numerous abscesses are found in the kidney.

Treatment: Supportive therapy is required; the diet should be well balanced, but not too high in protein. Vitamin supplementation is beneficial (Tx 22 and 23). If a suppurative nephritis is suspected antibiotics should be given (Tx 1–4).

THE DIGESTIVE SYSTEM

Malocclusion (slobbers)

This is one of the commonest conditions encountered in practice; however, it is generally at an advanced stage when the clinical signs become apparent, and the long term prognosis is usually poor.

The teeth grow continually through life at a rate of approximately 5–7.5 cm/year (2–3 inches/year), and their structure will be affected by changes in nutrition. The jaw moves both up and down, and from side to side during mastication. The rate of wear of the teeth should equal their rate of growth. The teeth are single rooted, which makes them more vulnerable to infection. Normal chinchilla teeth are yellow in colour; white teeth may indicate a vitamin A deficiency.

In malocclusion the teeth wear unevenly, causing overgrowth or uneven growth of the incisors, and spurs of tooth from the molars and premolars which may grow towards the tongue and the lips. As the condition progresses mastication becomes more uncomfortable and only soft foods are selectively eaten, resulting in further tooth growth as the chinchilla is no longer gnawing.

The tooth roots also grow through life. Often the earliest symptoms of malocclusion are lacrimal discharges as the upper tooth roots grow towards the orbit. The lower tooth roots grow down into the mandible; this can be palpated as a rough bumpy edge to the lower mandible. Some of the latter cases may not have uneven growth of the lower teeth tables, but suffer discomfort associated with the growth of the tooth roots similar to impacted wisdom teeth.

Malocclusion is in part hereditary, but diet and other oral conditions may also play an important part in its development. The onset of clinical signs may be up to 2 years, often after individuals have been used for breeding; however, once symptoms are obvious the affected animals should not be used.

Clinical signs: In the very early stages all that may be noticeable is an ocular discharge associated with the upper tooth roots impinging on the orbit. The incisors should be checked regularly for any sign of uneven wear or overgrowth. The upper incisors should be approximately 5 mm long, and the lower incisors 9 mm. Both sets of incisors are tapered to a point at the front. Any deviation in the incisors will indicate that the molars and premolars may start to wear unevenly.

As the condition progresses there may be a partial anorexia, the chinchilla selecting soft foods in preference to hard food. The droppings, once soft and round, become scant and smaller. As less food is eaten weight loss occurs. When the molar teeth become uncomfortable, or spurs of teeth begin to traumatise the tongue and cheeks the chinchilla will salivate profusely, and have a damp chest and forelegs. Mastication may become difficult, and often a grinding or clicking sound will be heard as the chinchilla tries to eat.

There may be pain on palpation of the upper jaw around the eyes associated with the upper tooth roots, in later stages the ocular discharge may be purulent.

Diagnosis: The incisors should be regularly inspected for signs of uneven wear. The molars and premolars can be inspected with an otoscope, or under sedation (such as a ketamine and acepromazine combination, using a dose of 40 mg/kg ketamine hydrochloride and 0.5 mg/kg acepromazine). The latter technique allows a more detailed inspection using a rodent mouth gag and pouch dilator, and clipping and filing can be undertaken. The mouth should be checked for the presence of foreign bodies between the teeth, or any infection which will also cause salivation, and these treated appropriately.

Radiographs of the head will detail the extent of the root growth, both into the orbit and the lower mandible. The frontal sinuses may appear to contain a pus like substance. The teeth may show a separation from the jaw bones, and the jawbones may appear thin and have a honeycomb appearance (other bones in the body may have a similar appearance).

Treatment: In the early stages the incisors can be trimmed, and plentiful hard food supplied to encourage gnawing and tooth wear. Pumice stone can be kept in the cage for gnawing. If the molar teeth have overgrown spurs, these can be trimmed and filed. Sedation with ketamine (at a dose of 40 mg/kg) plus acepromazine (0.5 mg/kg) given by intramuscular injection is ideal for restraint for dental work. The overgrown spurs may need to be filed every 6–8 weeks, and in the intervals between hard food should be offered. A calcium/vitamin D supplement (Tx 24. Collo-Cal D) may also be beneficial.

The prognosis is poor for very advanced cases, or in cases where the tables wear evenly, and the pain is associated with root overgrowth and impaction. These cases may be supported with the feeding of baby cereals, and steroid injections (Tx 9. Depomedrone) given intramuscularly for a while. Euthanasia should be considered.

Diet: Provision of a pumice stone or similar will encourage gnawing. Plenty of hay should be available to encourage mastication throughout the day because, although a pelleted ration may be hard and supply the recommended nutrients, the chinchilla will not take long to eat the day's ration and will then spend little of the rest of the day chewing. Herbivores by their nature should spend hours 'grazing' and chewing.

Too many soft treats should be avoided because these will be eaten selectively, and the chinchilla's appetite may be satisfied before it eats its staple ration.

The most important nutrients for the healthy formation of bones and teeth are calcium, phosphorus and vitamins A, D and B. The ratio of calcium:phosphorus should be between 1:1 and 2:1. The calcium requirements of the chinchilla are dynamic and depend upon its stage of life. Those of an adult female double during lactation; at this time attention to diet is extremely important, and supplementation with powdered milk or Bemax may be recommended. Sterilised bone meal or bone flour will provide calcium and phosphorus in the correct ratio of 2:1 and can be given at a maintenance rate of half a teaspoonful twice a week per adult.

Broken teeth

The incisor teeth may become broken as the result of a fall; they must be clipped and filed evenly so that malocclusion does not develop from uneven wear as the teeth grow back to the required length.

Mouth conditions

Foreign bodies, such as hay seeds or grass, may become lodged under the tongue or impacted in the cheeks, causing inflammation, infection and necrosis. Soft foods may become impacted around the teeth, or stuck on the roof of the mouth interfering with prehension. Examination of the mouth, if necessary under sedation, and removal of the foreign material is indicated. The areas of inflammation can be bathed with an antiseptic solution.

Unless detected early, such conditions will cause anorexia, salivation, and an overgrowth of the teeth resulting in slobbers.

The oesophagus (choke)

Occasionally a piece of foodstuff, or in youngsters a piece of bedding, may become lodged in the oesophagus. Initially the chinchilla may attempt to cough or retch up the obstruction, but unless intervention is rapid, death often occurs from suffocation. Choke may be responsible for the sudden death of previously fit individuals.

The stomach and intestines

Improper diets are responsible for many digestive disorders. The chinchilla requires a diet that is high in fibre, with moderate amounts of protein. Alterations to the diet must be introduced very gradually.

In common with other rodents, chinchillas are susceptible to antibiotic-induced diarrhoea caused by the use of narrow spectrum antibiotics against gram positive organisms. These allow proliferation of *Escherichia coli* and *Clostridia* spp. in the caecum causing a fatal enterotoxaemia.

Bloat

This occurs when there is a build up of gas in the stomach, often triggered by a change in diet, gastric stasis and fermentation by the bacterial flora. It is associated with a lack of *Bacillus acidophilus* (an acid forming organism usually present in the intestine). Bloat is commonest in hand fed or older animals.

Clinical signs: Usually 2 hours or more after feeding the abdomen becomes distended and affected animals show obvious abdominal discomfort by rolling and stretching. The pressure of the gas on the thorax causes dyspnoea.

Treatment: The gas must be relieved rapidly, either via a stomach tube, or by paracentesis. Liquid paraffin can be given orally (4–5 drops) to help the passage of ingesta and prevent further fermentation.

The pain can be managed with hyoscine (Tx 18. Buscopan compositum) at a dose of 0.2 ml by subcutaneous injection. Milpar (Tx 20) can be given to attempt to relieve the bloat. In the early stages increased exercise may be helpful, together with gentle massage of the abdomen.

Causes: The most common cause is the feeding of fruits and greens, which cause a decrease in the fibre intake and allow gastric fermentation to take place. Any fresh food must be offered sparingly and gradually.

Gastric distension and associated hind-limb paralysis may be seen in lactating females (see tympanites).

If bloat occurs in hand-fed young it may be necessary to feed them a more dilute mixture consisting of 30% evaporated milk, 60% boiled water and 10% glucose.

Gastric ulceration

Clinical signs: Anorexia and regurgitation are evident. Gastric ulceration is seen in young animals fed abrasive roughage or mouldy food.

Treatment: It is necessary to improve the diet, and the administration of gastric protectants, e.g. milk of magnesia (Tx 21) is indicated. Kaolin alone or in combination with pectin (Tx 19. Kaogel) can be given up to three times a day.

Intussusception

This may follow enteritis, or gastric tympany. It may also be associated with constipation and rectal prolapse. The chinchilla will show signs of colic, and the intussusception will be palpable. Surgical intervention is necessary.

Constipation

Clinical signs: There are scant hard droppings, often associated with a lack of fibre in the diet, or a reduced appetite for fibre secondary to malocclusion. A firm mass is palpable in the abdomen. The hind legs may appear uncoordinated or paralysed as the condition progresses. Other predisposing factors are lack of exercise, overcrowding, lack of water and stress. Constipation can occur in the female during the first week postpartum.

Treatment: Liquid paraffin, prune juice or syrup of figs can be given by mouth at a dose of 3–4 drops given three times daily. Up to 2 ml can be given daily. A few drops of milk of magnesia (Tx 21) could also be given. Alternatively, a solution of brown sugar dissolved in water can be given every 3–4 hours. Orange juice can be added to this solution to increase its palatability. If the chinchilla is eating, a diet of green foods, particularly dandelions and groundsel both of which are laxative, can be fed. Warm soapy enemas may be helpful in relieving the obstruction.

The chinchilla should be encouraged to exercise. More hay should be included in the daily ration.

Rectal prolapse

Clinical signs: This may follow constipation or diarrhoea because both cause increased abdominal straining. Initially the rectal mucosa may evert as the individual strains, and this may progress to a larger prolapse of rectal mucosa from the anus. The mucosa will be red and congested immediately after the prolapse occurs, becoming purple and necrotic with time.

Treatment: This should be effective if instigated early. The mucosa should be cleaned with an antiseptic solution, and it can be encouraged to shrink with a strong sugar solution applied to it. The prolapse can be returned by gentle manipulation with a thermometer. It may be useful to tighten the anal ring with a purse-string suture. Antibiotics (Tx 1–4) should be given post-operatively, and the chinchilla can be fed small amounts of pellets. Fibrous foods such as hay can be reintroduced after a few days. Glucose water or sugar in water is recommended for the first few days.

Diarrhoea

Diarrhoea associated with gastroenteritis may be bacterial, protozoal, parasitic or dietary in origin. Diarrhoea may also be induced by certain antibiotics. In each case the symptoms are similar, as are the principles of treatment.

Clinical signs: The diarrhoea is often watery and may contain blood or mucus. The chinchilla is dull, hunched, anorexic and lethargic. There may be pain on abdominal palpation. Continued abdominal straining or diarrhoea may lead to rectal prolapse.

Treatment: Fluid replacement is necessary, either with a proprietary brand (e.g. Lectade or Duphalyte) or warm water and glucose, flavoured with a little orange juice to increase its palatability. The normal bacteria of the gut should be repopulated with a probiotic such as Avipro (Tx 5), or with natural yogurt containing *Lactobacillus* spp. Alternatively, the digestive system can be repopulated with macerated droppings from a healthy chinchilla and given twice daily for 3–4 days.

Burnt toast, powdered arrowroot or arrowroot biscuits are also useful, and plenty of fibre in the form of good quality hay should be offered. The feeding of porridge oats instead of the normal rations for a few days will settle diarrhoea of dietary origin. A suspension containing kaolin and pectin (Tx 19. Kaogel) can be given at a dose of 4 drops three times a day. Hyoscine (Tx 18. Buscopan compositium) can be given at a dose of 0.2 ml by subcutaneous injection to control the abdominal pain.

Specific causes of enteritis

Bacterial

The normal gut flora consists of gram-positive bacteria, *Bifidobacterium* sp., *Bacteroides* spp., *Eubacterium* spp. and *Lactobacillus* spp. Enteritis is caused by *Escherichia coli*, *Proteus* spp., *Salmonella typhimurium*, *Pseudomonas*, *Corynebacterium* and *Yersinia*. *Listeria monocytogenes* will also produce symptoms of enteritis, as well as neurological symptoms of head tilt, circling and convulsions.

The pathogenic bacteria may be introduced by wild rodents, or by ingestion of contaminated feed. If left untreated the enteritis may progress to septicaemia, the bacteria spreading through the blood to many organs, particularly the liver and spleen. Affected individuals rapidly lose condition, and have rough dull fur. The diarrhoea is often associated with blood and mucus. Sudden death may be seen in associated animals.

Diagnosis: Culture and isolation of the bacterium from the blood, liver and spleen in the case of septicaemia are necessary to identify the organism in order to contain the spread of disease.

Treatment: Antibiotics must be used with care in order not to destroy the balance of normal gut flora further. Sulphonamides (Tx 4. Borgal 7.5%) can be given by subcutaneous injection, or neomycin can be given orally. A probiotic (Tx 5. Avipro) should be administered simultaneously.

Prophylactic antibiotics may be necessary to contain epizootics. Chloramphenicol (Tx 1) or oxytetracycline (Tx 3) are most frequently used for prophylactic therapy.

Protozoal

Healthy chinchillas may carry small numbers of several protozoa; however, increased numbers may cause enteritis. *Giardia*, *Trichomonas* spp., *Coccidia* and *Balantidium* spp. can all be found in moderate numbers. Stress, or concurrent infection may allow these protozoa to proliferate and cause disease.

Chinchillas infected with *Giardia* will have recurrent diarrhoea with no mucus, and will otherwise appear healthy.

Treatment: Metronidazole can be used. An adult chinchilla should receive 0.25 ml of Flagyl-s (Tx 26) daily given orally.

Parasitic

Nematodes and cestodes are also present in healthy chinchillas, but may cause enteritis if present in significant numbers. The commonest tapeworm is *Hymenolepis nana*.

Treatment: Fenbendazole is a suitable anthelmintic, and a 10% solution (Tx 27. Panacur) can be given orally at a dose of 0.5 ml/kg daily for 3 days.

Coprophagy

The eating of the softer caecotrophs is a normal part of the digestive process in the chinchilla. These softer caecal faeces contain B-complex vitamins which are formed in the caecum, and are an essential part of the chinchilla's diet.

Fatty liver

Fat deposits occur in the liver if an unsuitable diet is fed, particularly whole milk, peanuts, sunflower seeds and other 'pet' foods. Fatty liver is generally associated with obesity. Vitamin E deficiency will also cause fat to be deposited in the liver. Correction of the diet will improve the condition.

THE RESPIRATORY SYSTEM

Predisposing factors for the development of respiratory disease are over-crowding, poor ventilation, poor nutrition, a sudden change in temperature or humidity, or when the weather is cold and damp. Dusty atmospheres will also weaken the respiratory system's defence against infection. Young kits are particularly susceptible if they become damp or chilled. Cold and draughts must be avoided.

Some bacteria such as *Streptococcus* spp., *Pseudomonas* and *Pasteurella*, in small quantities make up the normal flora of the respiratory tract. In situations of stress they may proliferate in sufficient numbers to become pathogenic.

Inflammation of the nares

Inflammation may occur as a single entity, associated with slobbers, or as a precursor to upper respiratory tract infection. The affected chinchilla may rub its nose frequently; only occasionally is there a nasal discharge. Sometimes an affected chinchilla may die suddenly: this is because in some instances the infection damages the nasal sinuses and the inflammation leads to meningitis.

Treatment: Antibiotic therapy (Tx 1–4) will prevent the progression of infection. It may be useful to flush the nasal passages with antibiotic. The dust bath should be removed because the chinchilla is likely to persistently rub its face in the sand and the subsequent inhalation of sand particles may weaken the nasal passages further.

Upper respiratory tract infection

Clinical signs: The nares become inflamed. There may or may not be a nasal discharge in the early stages; however, a serous nasal discharge is a feature as the disease progresses. The affected chinchilla will sneeze, and young kits will shiver in an attempt to keep warm. There may also be an ocular discharge causing the eyelids to stick together. The fur on the inside of the front legs may become matted as the chinchilla rubs its wet nose. The disease may progress to pneumonia. The appetite is reduced.

It is suggested that humans with colds may be able to transmit the infection to chinchillas (Handbook of Rodent and Rabbit Medicine, p. 159).

Treatment: Supportive nursing is required, together with the provision of warmth and fluids. If an ocular discharge is present the eyes should be bathed gently with warm water and an antibiotic preparation applied (Tx 30–33). Antibiotics (Tx 1–4) should also be given by injection or orally. A little mentholated vapour ointment (e.g. Vick) can be applied around the cage to help clear the nasal passages. Alternatively, oil of eucalyptus and friar's balsam can be vaporised in the environment to help soothe and decongest the nasal passages. Pseudoephedrine hydrochloride solution (Tx. 29 Sudafed) can be given orally, at a dose of 0.2 ml/adult twice daily.

Vitamin supplementation (Tx 22 and 23) is useful to increase the resistance to infection.

Pneumonia

This may occur as a primary disease process, or as a progression from upper respiratory tract infection. Bacteria such as *Bordetella*, *Streptococcus* and *Pasteurella* are isolated in large numbers.

Clinical signs: Fever (up to 40–41°C (104–105°F)), lethargy, and laboured and shallow breathing are evident. The chest sounds are wheezy.

Treatment: In advanced cases treatment may be unsuccessful. Provision of warmth and dry surroundings is important. Antibiotics (Tx 1–4) should be given. Anti-inflammatory drugs can be given to manage the fever: 2 mg/kg ketofen can be given by subcutaneous injection, or paediatric paracetamol (e.g. Tx 28. Calpol) can be given at a dose of 100 mg/kg orally. It may be advisable to treat in-contact chinchillas with antibiotics prophylactically.

Inhalation pneumonia

This occurs particularly in hand-reared young when liquid may enter the trachea. It may also occur during improper administration of oral drugs.

Clinical signs: These are similar to those of infective pneumonia; laboured breathing and pyrexia are evident. Frothy bubbles may appear from the nostrils. Treatment is generally unrewarding.

Pleurisy

This may follow pneumonia, or occur as a result of trauma to the chest.

Clinical signs: There is chest pain, and associated stiff gait. The chinchilla sits hunched up with laboured breathing. Pyrexia (up to 41°C (105°F)), anorexia and polydipsia occur. The condition may progress to pyothorax.

Treatment: Mild cases should respond to antibiotics and supportive care; the provision of warmth is important. Any traumatic wounds to the outside of the chest should be cleaned with an antiseptic solution.

THE EYE

Ocular discharge

A serous ocular discharge may be associated with malocclusion, foreign bodies in the eye (e.g. sand, or seeds from poor quality hay), conjunctivitis, the onset of respiratory tract infection, or vitamin A deficiency.

The eyes should be examined for the presence of a foreign body, or any corneal abrasion; if present, the eye should be bathed with an antiseptic solution, and an antibiotic eye ointment or drops applied (Tx 30–33). Whilst any symptoms are present the sand bath should be removed to avoid further rubbing of the eye and possible damage. Conjunctivitis not accompanied by corneal abrasion can be treated with an antibiotic/steroid eye preparation (Tx 31 and 32).

Watery eyes may be the first indication of malocclusion, as the tooth roots of the upper pre-molars and molars extend towards the orbit. The teeth should be examined for any sign of abnormal wear (see Slobbers).

Vitamin A deficiency is associated with an ocular discharge, also dull hair coat, and reproductive disorders such as abortions and the birth of weak, blind young. It may be associated with the feeding of rancid cod-liver oil. Treatment requires the injection of vitamin A (2000 i.u.) daily for 7 days.

A purulent ocular discharge is associated with respiratory infection. The eyes must be bathed, and antibiotic ointment (Tx 30–32) applied. Antibiotics also need to be given orally, or by injection (Tx 1–4).

THE EAR

Chinchillas have very large, well developed tympanic bullae, and large thin pinnae. Their sense of hearing is acute.

Ear injuries

- *Trauma*. Bite wounds and subsequent tears are a sequel to fighting. The affected areas should be bathed with an antiseptic solution. Antibiotics (Tx 1–4) can be applied in an ointment, and given orally or by injection as necessary. To prevent further infection the sand bath should be removed whilst the ear is healing.
- *Infection*. Infections of the pinna may progress to middle ear infection if left untreated. It is important to maintain a patent ear canal and apply an aural preparation of antibiotics; any dog or cat preparation would be suitable. Systemic antibiosis (Tx 1–4) may be required. Inner ear infections are rare; a head tilt to the affected side is the presenting clinical sign. On radiographs the large tympanic bulla is seen to contain pus and debris. Treatment with antibiotics (Tx 1–4) may be effective. Drainage of the affected bulla could be considered. The sand bath should be removed whilst the chinchilla is undergoing treatment.
- *Haematoma*. Trauma may lead to the formation of an aural haematoma; the pinna becomes hard and painful as it fills up with blood. The haematoma should be drained, and if necessary stitched flat to prevent re-filling. Antibiotics should be given post-operatively.

Yellow ears

Clinical signs: The ears undergo a colour change to yellow and then orange. Other areas of the body, the abdomen and genitals may also become discoloured. Painful swellings may occur on the abdomen.

Chinchillas require adequate amounts of choline, methionine and vitamin E in the diet so that the liver is able to break down plant pigments such as carotene. If there are inadequate amounts of any of these, the plant pigments become deposited in the fat and skin.

Treatment: Supplementation of the diet with adequate amounts of choline, methionine and vitamin E.

THE MUSCULOSKELETAL SYSTEM

Fractures

Simple fractures of the long bones can be repaired by internal fixation, using a needle as an intramedullary pin. Comminuted or compound fractures may require amputation. Chinchillas have a tendency to chew at the injured leg, and may need to wear an Elizabethan collar whilst healing is in progress. Fractures heal quickly, with callous formation taking place within 7–10 days.

Tail injuries

Tail injuries occur if the tail is grasped at its end, resulting in a degloving of the tip of the tail. Small injuries may heal with the application of antiseptic wound powder; larger injuries may require amputation.

MISCELLANEOUS CONDITIONS

Heat stroke

Chinchillas are particularly susceptible to heat stroke, and will become easily distressed at temperatures above 25°C. This is compounded if the humidity is also high. Chinchillas should never be placed in direct sunlight, or near a radiator. If they are kept in an outdoor building it may help to paint the roof white, because this will reflect the sunlight and keep the building cool. The condition may also occur during transportation. If animals are transported in the heat, it is useful to provide a freezer ice pack to help prevent heat prostration.

Obese animals are most usually affected, but heat stroke may occur after periods of increased activity, e.g. mating or using the sand bath. For these reasons it is a sensible precaution to offer the sand bath in the coolest part of the day during summer.

Clinical signs: In the initial stages the chinchilla will be restless and polydipsic. As it becomes further affected it will lie on its side and become dyspnoeic, mouth breathing becoming evident. The lungs become congested, and haemorrhagic frothy fluid may appear at the mouth and nostrils.

Treatment: Affected animals must be handled very carefully to avoid further stress. The individual should be cooled slowly by immersion in lukewarm water and placed in a cool, well ventilated area. Alternatively the chinchilla can be wrapped in a damp towel. A respiratory stimulant such as etamiphylline (Tx 16. Millophyline) can be given by subcutaneous injection, and a short acting corticosteroid (Tx 7 and 8) may also be useful. Cool water can be given by dropper in the later stages of recovery.

Fits

Fits may occur after eating, and are usually associated with an acute colic. This may be triggered by eating cold food. Excess exercise, calcium or vitamin B deficiencies, or toxic infections resulting in meningitis may all also cause convulsions.

Treatment: Colic fits can be treated with a subcutaneous injection of 0.2 ml hyoscine (Tx 18. Buscopan compositum). Dietary deficiencies can be corrected with vitamin B injections (Tx 23), and the addition of bone meal to the diet. Calcium gluconate can be given by intraperitoneal injection at a dose of 100 mg/kg.

Anorexia

The appetite can be stimulated by the administration of a probiotic (Tx 5) or with foods such as apples, raisins and prunes. These fruits are also a good source of B vitamins and trace minerals.

3 ANAESTHESIA AND DRUG TREATMENTS

HANDLING

Chinchillas are docile creatures and easy to handle. Rough handling must be avoided as they will shed patches of fur; this is known as fur slip. They can either be picked up with a hand around their shoulders, or grasped by the tail base with one hand, the other supporting the body.

NURSING

Provision of warmth and comfort is important for the chinchilla. Warmth can be provided via a heating pad, an infra red lamp, or young orphans can be placed in a box in an airing cupboard.

PRE-ANAESTHETIC PREPARATION

Food and water need not be withheld before surgery, because the chinchilla is unable to vomit. Dehydration will potentiate the effects of any anaesthetic, and if the patient has not been drinking some pre-operative fluid replacement may be necessary. Fluids can be given subcutaneously, at a rate of 10 ml/kg body weight.

It is important to weigh the patient accurately for the calculation of dose rates, and small quantities of drugs should be given in an insulin syringe.

If an inhalation anaesthetic is used the chinchilla should receive a pre-medication with atropine at a dose of 0.05 mg/kg. For surgical procedures an inhalation agent is most suitable.

One of the major problems of surgery is the potential for heat loss during the procedure. This can be minimised by placing the patient on a heat-reflective surface, e.g. Flectabed, or by wrapping the patient in aluminium foil. Heat can also be provided by a heat lamp above the operating table. A hot water bottle should not be used because it will encourage vasodilation, and increase heat loss further.

If surgery is to be carried out, the operation site should be clipped, and cleaned with an antibacterial agent, e.g. a povidone-iodine solution. The cleaning solution should be warmed to body temperature, and used sparingly so as not to cause heat loss through evaporation. The surgical site should then be sprayed with surgical spirit.

ANAESTHESIA

Inhalation anaesthesia

An inhalation agent is best for surgical procedures and this can be administered through a face mask. Halothane or isoflurane are both suitable for this.

Dose: Induction with either halothane or isoflurane can be achieved using a 3% concentration, with the anaesthesia maintained with a lower concentration of 1–2%. This can be used with oxygen alone, or a 1:1 mixture of oxygen and nitrous oxide.

Injection anaesthesia

For inspection of teeth and dental work an injectable combination is recommended. The combination of ketamine hydrochloride and acepromazine provides excellent restraint. The patient should be weighed accurately to calculate the dose of the drugs, and an insulin syringe used for administering them.

Dose: The dose is 40 mg/kg of ketamine hydrochloride and 0.5 mg/kg acepromazine. The drugs can be mixed in the same syringe and given by intramuscular injection. The injection should be given into the quadriceps muscle using a 23–25 gauge needle.

ANALGESIA

Analgesia is useful post-operatively, and in any other instance of pain.

Buprenorphine (Vetergesic, Animalcare Ltd.)

Dose: This can be given at a dose of 0.05 mg/kg by subcutaneous injection every 8–12 hours. Vetergesic contains 0.3 mg/ml buprenorphine and a dose for an adult chinchilla would be 0.08–0.1 ml.

Carprophen (Zenecarp, C-Vet)

Dose: This can be given at a dose of 4 mg/kg. Zenecarp injection contains 50 mg/ml carprophen, and a dose for an average adult chinchilla is 0.04 ml by subcutaneous injection. Zenecarp is best given pre-operatively, and a single dose lasts 24 hours.

POST-OPERATIVE CARE

The chinchilla should recover in a temperature of 35°C (95°F), and then maintained in an environment of 20–25°C (68–77°F) for the next 24 hours. Recovery can be made on a vetbed or a heat-reflective surface, e.g. Flectabed, so that the patient keeps warm and dry. The patient must be dried if it passes urine, so that the urine does not soak into the coat and cause hypothermia. The environment should be as stress-free as possible.

If the surgery has resulted in a sutured wound, the patient should be kept on a towel or vetbed to protect the wound whilst healing, and no sandbaths must be given until the wound has healed.

The patient should be encouraged to eat and drink, and if necessary should be fed through an eye dropper, or syringe. Human baby cereals are ideal, to which can be added a probiotic (Tx 5) to help maintain the gut flora and stimulate the appetite.

Fluid replacement therapy

Fluids should be given either intra-operatively, or post-operatively. Warmed glucose-saline (0.9% saline, 5% glucose) is suitable and 5–10 ml can be given subcutaneously.

DRUG TREATMENTS

Antibiotics

Antibiotics can be administered by injection or orally. They can be given in the drinking water, but it is important to take into consideration that a sick animal may drink less, or not at all. Oral medicines can be administered via an eye dropper, or concealed in a treat such as a raisin.

Antibiotic therapy must be chosen with care, because the action of some antibiotics will alter the normal gut flora and allow the intestines to become colonised with *Clostridium* spp. which cause a fatal enterotoxaemia. The most toxic drugs are those with a narrow spectrum of action against Gram-positive organisms, especially penicillin and its derivatives, lincomycin, clindamycin and erythromycin. Broad spectrum antibiotics are a little safer, but none are totally free from the risk of inducing this condition, and it is advisable to administer a probiotic at the same time as dosing with anti-biotics. Concurrent administration of a vitamin supplement (Tx 22 and 23) is also recommended, because during a period of illness and antibiotic administration the uptake of vitamins in the gut is likely to be upset.

Tx 1. Chloramphenicol

Chloramphenicol '100' tablets (Willows Francis Ltd.)

These tablets contain 100 mg chloramphenicol PhEur.

Dose: 50 mg/kg orally twice daily. For an average adult one quarter of a tablet can be crushed and administered orally twice a day.

Tx 2. Enrofloxacin

Baytril (Bayer plc)

This is a broad spectrum bactericidal antibiotic, which is now the preferred drug for most infections.

Dose: 5–10mg/kg daily.
The 2.5% injection solution can be given subcutaneously at a dose of 0.3 ml/kg daily. The 2.5% oral solution can be diluted 1:1 with blackcurrant syrup and given orally. An adult dose would be 0.2 ml of the mixture twice

daily. The 5% injection solution can be mixed with the drinking water to give a dose of 200 mg/litre. This can be achieved by taking 4 ml of the 5% injection solution and making it up to 1 litre with water.

Tx 3. Oxytetracycline

Oxycare Tablets (Animalcare Ltd.)

These each contain 50 mg oxytetracycline.

Dose: 50–100 mg/kg orally twice daily. The tablets can conveniently be crushed.

Tx 4. Potentiated sulphonamides

Borgal 7.5% (Hoechst UK Ltd.)

This contains 12.5 mg/ml trimethoprim and 62.5 mg/ml sulphadoxine.

Dose: 0.5 ml/kg daily by subcutaneous injection (average adult dose 0.3 ml).

Tribrissen 24% Injection (Mallinckrodt Veterinary Ltd.)

This contains 40 mg/ml trimethoprim and 200 mg/ml sulphadiazine.

Dose: The injection can be diluted 1–2 ml into 1 litre of water, and used as medicated drinking water.

Probiotics

Probiotics contain a supply of beneficial bacteria to help colonise the gastrointestinal tract. They are useful for protecting the gut flora during antibiotic administration, and can also be given to help stimulate the appetite, or used in times of stress.

Tx 5. Avipro (Vetark Health)

This contains *Lactobacillus acidophilus, Enterococcus faecium, Saccharomyces* and electrolytes.

Dose: 5 gm is dissolved in 200 ml drinking water.

Antifungal agents

Tx 6. Griseofulvin

Grisovin Tablets (Mallinckrodt Veterinary Ltd.)

The tablets each contain 125 mg griseofulvin.

Dose: An adult may be given 25 mg/kg twice daily or 50 mg/kg daily for at least a month; one eighth of a tablet can be given twice daily or one quarter of a tablet every day.

Corticosteroids

There are several different corticosteroid preparations available, each with a different speed of action and duration of therapeutic value. Steroids are contraindicated in pregnancy because they may cause fetal abnormalities, and their use in late pregnancy may cause early parturition or abortion.

Tx 7. Betamethasone

Betsolan injection (Mallinckrodt Veterinary Ltd.)

This contains 2 mg/ml betamethasone, and is a powerful anti-inflammatory.

Dose: 0.1–0.2 ml may be given by subcutaneous or intramuscular injection.

Tx 8. Dexamethasone

Dexafort (Intervet UK Ltd.)

This is a combination of long- and short-acting steroids which produces a rapid and long-lasting glucogenic effect, and a long anti-inflammatory and anti-pruritic effect.

Dose: 0.1 ml may be given by subcutaneous or intramuscular injection.

Tx 9. Methylprednisolone

Depomedrone V (Upjohn Ltd.)

This contains 40 mg/ml methylprednisolone with a therapeutic action that lasts from 1–4 weeks.

Dose: Up to 0.2 ml may be given by intramuscular injection.

Miscellaneous treatments

Tx 10. Atropine

Atropine sulphate injection BP (Vet) 600 µg/ml

Dose: 50 µg/kg (0.05 mg/kg). For an average adult this requires 0.025–0.05 ml to be given by subcutaneous injection.

Tx 11. Bromhexine hydrochloride

Bisolvon (Boehringer Ingelheim)

This is a mucolytic which is a useful adjunct to the treatment of respiratory disease.

Dose: The injection solution contains 3 mg/ml bromohexine and 0.2 ml can be given to an adult daily by subcutaneous injection. The powder contains 10 mg/g bromhexine hydrochloride and 0.1 g (a small pinch) can be given twice daily.

Tx 12. Pyrethrin

Anti-mite Spray for Birds (Johnson)

This contains 0.8% w/v pyrethrin and 1% w/v piperonyl butoxide BP.

Dose: A light spray may be given and repeated weekly if necessary.

Tx 13. Chamomile

Kamillosan (Norgine Ltd.)

This ointment contains 10.5% w/v chamomile. It is particularly useful in the treatment of sore nipples and is safe even when the young are suckling.

Dose: A little can be applied to the affected nipples two or three times daily.

Tx 14. Dermisol (Pfizer Ltd.)

This is a topical preparation which contains propylene glycol, malic acid, benzoic acid and salicylic acid. It promotes healing by removing dead and necrotic tissue from affected areas and also has antibacterial properties. It can be applied two or three times daily.

Tx 15. Hexachlorophane

Ster-zac Powder (Houghs Healthcare Ltd.)

This contains 0.33% hexachlorophane, 3% zinc oxide and sterilised talc. It is effective in preventing staphylococcal infections.

Tx 16. Etamiphylline

Millophyline-V Injection (Arnolds Veterinary Products)

This contains 140 mg/ml etamiphylline camsylate and is a cardiac and respiratory stimulant. It can be used alongside an antibiotic to treat respiratory infections, and is a useful supportive therapy for heat prostration.

Dose: 0.1 ml given by intramuscular or subcutaneous injection. The dose can be repeated up to three times daily as required.

Tx 17. Flunixin

Finadyne Injection (Schering-Plough Animal Health)

The injection contains 10 mg/ml flunixin meglumine, and is a potent non-steroidal, non-narcotic analgesic with anti-inflammatory, anti-endotoxic and anti-pyretic properties.

Dose: 1 mg/kg given by subcutaneous injection. For pain relief a single dose should be given daily. In cases of endotoxic shock the dose can be repeated after 12 hours.

Tx 18. Hyoscine N-butylbromide

Buscopan Compositum (Boehringer Ingelheim Ltd.)

This is a spasmolytic and analgesic, which is particularly useful for the treatment of gastrointestinal disorders and colic.

Dose: The injection, which contains 4 mg/ml hyoscine, can be give at a dose of 0.2 ml by subcutaneous injection to an adult twice daily. The tablets, containing 10 mg hyoscine, can be crushed and a quarter of a tablet given orally twice daily.

Tx 19. Kaolin

There are various preparations containing kaolin alone, or kaolin in combination with pectin.

Kaogel (Parke, Davis & Co. Ltd.)

This contains light kaolin 20% w/v and pectin 0.43% w/v and can be given at a dose of 0.2 ml three times daily.

Tx 20. Milpar

This contains 75% milk of magnesia and 25% liquid paraffin; the latter is useful when an additional laxative effect is required.

Dose: Up to 0.3 ml may be given two or three times daily.

Tx 21. Milk of magnesia

This contains 83 mg/ml magnesium hydroxide.

Dose: Up to 0.2 ml may be given orally two or three times daily.

Tx 22. Multivitamin preparations

Abidec Drops (Parke Davis)

These contain vitamins A, B_1 (thiamine), B_2, B_6, niacin, C and D. They can be given by mouth, or added to the water bottle.

Dose: Two or three drops daily are required for an adult, 2 drops for a youngster, and a single drop can be added to the mixture used for hand rearing.

Tx 23. Vitamin B$_{12}$

This is a very useful vitamin for use in convalescence, and in cases of debilitation or inappetance.

Dose: 0.2 ml of vitamin B$_{12}$ 240 µg can be given by subcutaneous injection, and this dose can be repeated weekly.

Tx 24. Calcium supplementation

Collo-Cal D (C-Vet)

This contains 0.75% w/v colloidal calcium oleate and 70 i.u./ml vitamin D.

Dose: 0.5 ml/kg may be given orally daily.

Tx 25. Primidone

Mysoline (Mallinckrodt Veterinary Ltd.)

The suspension contains 50 mg/ml primidone. It can be used to stabilise seizures of any origin.

Dose: 0.5 mg/kg may be given orally twice daily.

Tx 26. Metronidazole

Flagyl-s (May and Baker Ltd.)

This contains 40 mg/ml metronidazole and is effective against protozoa.

Dose: 20 mg/kg/day. An adult chinchilla should receive 0.25 ml per day given orally.

Tx 27. Fenbendazole

Panacur (Hoechst UK Ltd.)

This contains 10% fenbendazole, and is a suitable anthelmintic.

Dose: 0.5 ml/kg may be given daily for 3 days.

Tx 28. Paracetamol

Calpol (Wellcome Ltd.)

The six plus suspension of Calpol contains 50 mg/ml paracetamol. This may be useful in cases of pneumonia. In other instances where pain relief is necessary, Zenecarp is advised (p. 42).

Dose: 100 mg/kg may be given orally up to twice a day.

Tx 29. Pseudoephedrine hydrochloride

Sudafed (Wellcome Ltd.)

This human decongestant contains 6 mg/ml pseudoephedrine hydro-chloride.

Dose: 0.2 ml/adult may be given orally twice daily.

Eye preparations

These can be divided into two groups, antibiotic only and antibiotic/steroid combinations. The antibiotic content should be broad-spectrum as there is some risk of causing endotoxaemia if the chinchilla ingests the ointment during the grooming process, and broad spectrum antibiotics are considered the safest.

Whilst using eye medication the sandbaths should be witheld to prevent the chinchilla rubbing its eyes in the sand and exacerbating the original condition.

Tx 30. Cepravin Eye Ointment (Mallinckrodt Veterinary Ltd.)

This contains a semisynthetic broad-spectrum bactericidal cephalosporin. It can be applied once daily.

Tx 31. Neobiotic HC (Upjohn Ltd.)

This contains the antibiotic neomycin and hydrocortisone as the steroid. It is a ready flowing liquid and can be applied two or three times daily.

Tx 32. Maxitrol (Alcon Ltd.)

This contains an antibiotic (neomycin), steroid (dexamethasone), and an antifungal agent (polymyxin B). It can be applied two or three times daily.

Tx 33. Golden Eye Ointment (Typharm Ltd)

This is available from pharmacists and contains dibromopropamidine ise-thionate 0.15% w/w and liquid paraffin. It is useful for minor eye infections and conjunctivitis. It can be applied once or twice daily.

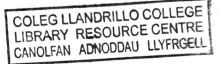

CHIPMUNKS

Chipmunks are members of the squirrel family, and they are classed between the tree squirrels and the ground-dwelling squirrels (e.g. the Prairie dog). They are found naturally in North America and Eurasia; the commonest species kept in captivity is the Siberian chipmunk, *Eutamius sibericus*. They are diurnal animals and live in burrows. In some areas of Siberia they will hibernate over winter, whilst in others they will remain active in their burrows, appearing at the surface when it is dry and mild. They are active climbers, and may make their nests in the hollows of trees.

4 HUSBANDRY AND NUTRITION

Housing

Chipmunks can be kept in a cage indoors, in a shed, or in a bird aviary. The cage size should be as large as possible, with a minimum height of 1.2 m. Chipmunks are avid gnawers, so the cage should be made of strong wire with fine mesh (2.5 cm × 2.5 cm) to prevent escape and also to prevent wild vermin entering. The base of the cage should be solid or made of wire and be capable of retaining the burrowing medium (see below). Outside cages and aviaries must be provided with adequate shelter, and must have a covered roof to prevent contamination by bird droppings.

One nest box must be provided for each chipmunk in the cage. These should be at least 15 cm × 20 cm × 15 cm, and larger for a breeding female. Inadequate provision of nest boxes will result in fighting. The nest boxes can be hung on the side of the cage and filled with good quality meadow hay, or other edible bedding for rodents; shredded paper and dry non-poisonous leaves are also suitable. Synthetic fibres should not be used because, like the hamster, the chipmunk may pouch the bedding, resulting in impaction if it is swallowed.

Branches such as apple and pear, which are safe to chew, should be provided for climbing and gnawing.

The base of the cage should be covered in a deep layer (10 cm or greater) of material for burrowing. One of the best combinations is peat, meadow hay and bark chippings or wood shavings, the proportions of which can vary depending on what is available. Plastic pipes can be added for variation.

Hibernation

Chipmunks kept outside will hibernate over winter, and must be provided with shelter, extra nesting material and plentiful stores of food. Their nest must be in a frost-proof position. When they hibernate their body temperature drops from 38°C (100°F), to a few degrees above the environmental temperature.

Some individuals may remain in the nest boxes on cold days, but emerge and become active if it becomes warmer.

Before hibernation members of the colony, particularly dominant males, may become more aggressive towards each other as they gather their food stores and injuries may occur.

Individuals which hibernate tend to have a shorter life span than those which remain active during the winter.

Hygiene

Cleaning is best done at night. The outside area only needs to be cleaned monthly, but the places used as latrines should be cleaned weekly. The nest boxes should also be cleaned out monthly during the spring and summer, and when a litter is weaned. In addition to cleaning fresh bedding should be added and some of the store of food replaced. However, in the autumn before the hibernation period the nest boxes should be left alone; they should be cleaned again in the spring.

Stocking

Chipmunks can be kept singly, in breeding pairs, or in groups of 3–5, with one male to 2–3 females. Single sex groups can also be kept together, although they may start fighting if there is limited space or there are insufficient nest boxes.

Adult chipmunks are difficult to tame, but youngsters, if hand reared or acquired before 8–16 weeks of age, may become very tame.

Nutrition

In the wild the chipmunk is omnivorous, eating a diet of seeds and berries, and also fruit, vegetables, grubs, birds' eggs and occasionally bird chicks.

In captivity the diet should be as balanced as possible. Dry mixes formulated for chipmunks are now available, or hamster mixes are a close approximation. These can be supplemented with fruits and vegetables such as cabbage, kale and carrots. Peaches and plums may be given, but their stones should be removed because they may be toxic. Wild plants such as dandelions, chickweed and shepherd's purse can be fed as long as they are well washed. Hard-boiled eggs, mealworms and tinned dog food can also be given. Wheat and wheatgerm are excellent sources of vitamin E, an increase of which in the diet improves fertility.

The diet of pregnant females can be supplemented with extra protein, milk powder, day old chicks, and hard-boiled eggs.

The eating of soft faecal pellets (coprophagy) is normal and essential for chipmunks to meet their vitamin requirements.

The dry mix should be given in solid heavy containers which cannot be tipped over. Chipmunks should be fed twice daily, in the morning and evening. Water should be provided from sipper bottles with stainless steel spouts, because chipmunks are able to chew through aluminium. If necessary vitamin supplements can be added in the drinking water.

The average food intake of an adult is 25–30 g daily, and much of the surplus food will be carried in the pouches to the food store, which is often in the nest box. This store should be checked daily for any fresh food which may become mouldy and cause digestive upsets. The food store should never be completely removed because it may encourage the chipmunk to keep food permanently in its cheek pouches, with subsequent damage to the pouches.

Problems associated with diet

- *Flaked maize.* An excess of this in the diet, particularly in the summer, may lead to overheating and pruritis.
- *Sunflower seeds.* These can be given as a treat. However, because they are high in fat and low in calcium an excess will lead not only to obesity and infertility, but also to calcium deficiency and bone fragility.
- *Overgrown incisors.* Chipmunks are constantly gnawing, and must be provided with adequate hard food to chew to prevent tooth overgrowth. The diet should be supplemented with hard food such as dog biscuits, unsweetened crackers or toast.

5 SYSTEMS AND DISEASES

THE SKIN

Abscesses

These occur most commonly after fighting, or from wounds that are caused by sharp edges of the cage or cage contents. Small clean cuts should heal without intervention, but where possible all wounds should be bathed with a mild antiseptic or saline solution. However, where the wound is small, and the chipmunk is unused to being handled, it is best left to heal on its own.

Treatment: If the wound becomes infected it should be cleaned and antibiotics given. It is easiest to isolate the chipmunk and medicate the water with antibiotics.

Prevention: It is important to remove any stress factors such as over-crowding, and ensure that there are enough nest boxes for each chipmunk to have its own. Aggression may increase in the autumn prior to hiber-nation as the chipmunks start food gathering.

Care must be taken when introducing any new chipmunk into a group; initially it is best put in a small cage inside the big cage to allow familiar-isation before it is released.

Tail-slip

Fighting or poor handling can easily result in a de-gloving injury to the tail. The damaged portion may dry and fall off without treatment, or may require surgical intervention.

Ectoparasites

Clinical signs: Alopecia, and pruritus. Fleas, harvest mites and burrowing mites can be found on chipmunks.

Treatment: Dusting with a pyrethrin powder, or spraying with fipronil (Tx 10. Frontline) at a dose rate of 7.5 mg/kg may be carried out.

If burrowing mites are suspected the chipmunk can be given 1 drop of 1% ivermectin solution by mouth (Tx 7. Ivomec Cattle Injection) and this can be repeated every 10 days.

Alopecia

Non-specific alopecia may be seen if there is a dietary imbalance. This should be corrected, and a small drop of unsaturated fatty acids (e.g. evening primrose oil) can be added to the food daily.

Alopecia that is accompanied by pruritus can be treated with steroid injections; dexamethasone (Tx 6. Dexafort) can be given.

THE REPRODUCTIVE SYSTEM

- Litter size: 1–8 (average 4)
- Birth weight: 3 g
- Weaning age: 40 days (one week after emergence from nest box)
- Fur grows: 14 days
- Eyes open: 14 days
- Breeding life of female: 1–6 years
- Breeding life of male: his lifetime 2–5 years
- Puberty: 8–14 months
- Oestrus: every 14 days
- Oestrus length: 3 days
- Gestation: 28–35 days

Sexing

The anogenital distance is greater in the male than the female. During the breeding season the male's testes will be visible in the scrotum; during the winter the testes will be retracted, but the penis will still be visible.

Females possess four pairs of mammary glands.

Breeding

The chipmunk is a seasonal breeder, and breeds from spring to autumn with peaks of activity in spring and mid-summer. In spring the male's testes descend into the scrotum; they retract in the autumn. Breeding is governed by climate and daylength; paradoxically, if daylight hours are extended artificially this may increase infertility.

Pairing and mating

The females generally come into season 2 weeks after the male's testes descend. The female's oestrus lasts 3 days, during which time she will call to the male in loud 'chips'. The pair generally mate on the second day of oestrus. If the male is only paired with the female at breeding time, she should be introduced into his cage and not vice versa. If necessary she can be placed in a small wire cage inside the male's cage to allow the pair to smell each other and get used to one another before she is released. A female would only accept a male in her cage on the second day of oestrus.

Gestation and post-partum care

Pregnant and lactating females may be best housed alone.

The young are born in the nest box, naked and blind. They are very vocal for the first 14 days of their life, at the end of which time they are furred and their eyes open. They emerge from the nest box around 30–38 days of age. In the wild the litter may stay together for another 6–8 weeks after leaving the nest, but in captivity they can be weaned between 6 and 8 weeks of age.

Most chipmunks rear one litter a year, but weaning this litter at 7 weeks can encourage the birth of a second litter, which is usually less prolific.

The nest box should be cleaned thoroughly after weaning.

Problems after parturition

Metritis

If a fetus is retained metritis is a likely sequel, leading to a noxious vaginal discharge, and often peritonitis. It is generally fatal.

Pyometra has also been recorded.

Hypocalcaemia

This may occur in nursing females, and can be corrected by feeding calcium rich foods such as milk, milk powder and cheese, or by adding a calcium supplement to the food, e.g. Collo-Cal D (Tx 8) at a dose of 0.1 ml daily.

Hand rearing

Hand rearing is possible if the young are aged a week or over, and will result in very tame individuals. A mixture of evaporated milk diluted 1:2 with boiled water should be fed initially, and after a week this can be thickened to a pouring consistency with baby cereal and be fed through a syringe or dropper. Glucose powder (5 g) and a probiotic, e.g. Avipro (Tx 4) (5 g) can be added to 200 ml of the hand-rearing mixture. For the first 1–2 weeks of life the young should be fed every 4 hours, then every 6 hours until 3 weeks of age when they can be fed three times daily. Care must be taken not to force the feed into the mouth and cause inhalation pneumonia; for this reason a small insulin syringe is useful. It is important to stimulate defaecation and urination after every feed by massaging the anogenital area with cotton wool soaked in warm water.

Infertility

- *Day length*. Although breeding is governed by photoperiod, an extended day length may actually reduce fertility. Chipmunks kept indoors may be exposed to too much light.
- *Stress*. It is important to provide breeding pairs with plenty of space and an adequate number of nest boxes. If they are cramped they will fail to breed.

  Other external influences which chipmunks find stressful are television sets, and the smells of other animals, particularly other rodents.

THE URINARY SYSTEM

Cystitis

Clinical signs: Haematuria, dysuria and loss of appetite are seen. Vomiting may also occur. The cystitis may result from a bacterial infection, but may also be associated with urolithiasis (usually struvite uroliths are found).

Treatment: If appropriate, urine analysis should be carried out and antibiotic treatment (Tx 1–3) given.

THE DIGESTIVE SYSTEM

Overgrown incisors

The teeth grow constantly through life, and adequate opportunity must be given for gnawing with an adequate supply of wood, dog biscuits, nuts, etc. If too much soft food is fed the teeth will overgrow, and the lower incisors may start to irritate the nares.

The teeth can be clipped, under anaesthesia should this be necessary if the chipmunk is not used to being handled. More hard foods should be added to the diet. The teeth may need to be clipped regularly, and if this is a stressful procedure, incisor extraction under anaesthesia could be considered.

Occasionally the jaw and teeth may become misaligned as the result of a fall or fight, requiring regular tooth clipping. This can only be done if it does not stress the chipmunk, otherwise euthanasia should be a considered alternative.

Dental caries

Dental caries are common in chipmunks fed a high carbohydrate or high acid diet. Salivation and dysphagia may also occur if a foreign body becomes lodged between the teeth, and it may be necessary to examine the mouth under anaesthesia.

STOMACH AND INTESTINES

Diarrhoea

Diarrhoea of dietary origin

The commonest cause of diarrhoea is a sudden dietary change, or the overfeeding of vegetables. If fresh food is stored in the food stores and allowed to decay this may also lead to digestive upset.

Nursing females may produce softer faeces, but this is normal.

Treatment: If the diarrhoea is the result of a change of food, the affected chipmunk should be given no fresh food, just hay and dry mix. Apple peel, burnt toast and raspberry or blackberry leaves are all astringent and can be offered. Powdered arrowroot can be sprinkled on the dry food.

Diarrhoea resulting from bacterial enteritis

Bacterial enteritis can also cause diarrhoea. Wild rodents such as mice can transmit *Salmonella* spp. which may be associated with diarrhoea and loss of condition.

Treatment: Antibiosis, with oxytetracycline, enrofloxacin or sulphonamides (Tx 1–3) should be given, along with dietary modification.

Constipation

Causes: This generally occurs due to the ingestion and impaction of unsuitable bedding material such as cotton wool, kapok or newspaper.

Clinical signs: The chipmunk may exhibit abdominal discomfort and bloating.

Treatment: Good quality hay should be offered, and plentiful moist fresh food. One or two drops of cod-liver oil can be added to the food to help ease the constipation.

THE RESPIRATORY SYSTEM

Pneumonia

Poor husbandry, particularly damp housing and overcrowding, predisposes to the development of pneumonia. Chipmunks can contract human influenza viruses if they are in contact with infected humans. The disease is usually fatal.

Clinical signs: The affected animal adopts a hunched posture; the respiratory rate is increased and there is anorexia.

Treatment: Affected chipmunks must be isolated in a clean, warm and well ventilated hospital cage. Antibiotics (Tx 2. oxytetracycline) can be given via the drinking water. Mentholated ointment, e.g. Vick, can be put near the cage.

Rhinitis

Clinical signs: Epistaxis, face rubbing and washing, and upper respiratory tract stridor are evident.

These signs may be due to overgrown incisors, or tooth decay associated with foreign bodies in the mouth, which should be treated appropriately.

THE EYE

Corneal ulceration and ocular discharge

Causes: Corneal ulceration and ocular discharge are generally caused by abrasions from bedding material, or through fighting.

Treatment: When possible the eye should be bathed with water or a mild saline solution and an appropriate antibiotic eye ointment used, preferably one that needs to be applied only once daily to reduce the stress of treatment (e.g. Tx 9. Orbenin Ophthalmic Ointment).

Cataracts

Cataracts and subsequent loss of vision are seen in older animals, particularly males, and it is thought that they may be hereditary. Affected animals may be able to cope adequately in a smaller cage with few obstacles.

THE MUSCULOSKELETAL SYSTEM

Fractures

Fractures may heal with conservative treatment; where possible it is better not to apply dressings because these are likely to initiate self-trauma and further injury. Severe fractures can be treated by amputation, which appears to be well accepted by the chipmunk.

Chipmunks may catch their digits in the cage wire, these will generally slough and heal without treatment.

MISCELLANEOUS CONDITIONS

Cage paralysis

Cage paralysis is thought to occur as the result of vitamin E deficiency, but it may also be a symptoms of myositis, toxoplasmosis, traumatic injury, or inner ear infection.

Clinical signs: Stiffness and reluctance to move, dragging of hind-quarters.

Treatment: Balanced diets should be fed; extra wheatgerm (a rich source of vitamin E) can be sprinkled on the dry food.

Fits

Epilepsy has been reported in chipmunks, as have both bacterial and viral meningitis.

6 ANAESTHESIA AND DRUG TREATMENTS

HANDLING

Adult chipmunks usually resist handling and bite! Hand reared animals, or individuals that have been handled from an early age may be tamed, and will sit in a cupped hand, or allow themselves to be held by the scruff of the neck.

Chipmunks can be caught in a butterfly net, or shut in a nest box for transportation. When trying to net them care must be taken not to chase them for too long, as any chase is stressful and exhausting.

It may be necessary to examine fractious patients under anaesthesia, and the nest box can become an anaesthetic chamber, and anaesthesia induced with halothane.

When handling chipmunks care must be taken not to grasp the tail, which will deglove easily. If this does occur the end of the tail should dry up and fall off, or become chewed off.

PRE-ANAESTHETIC PREPARATION

Pre-anaesthetic starvation is unnecessary as regurgitation cannot occur due to the anatomy of the cardia of the stomach. Water should also remain available as any restriction can exaggerate the metabolic effects of anaesthesia.

The patient must be accurately weighed to enable any drug doses to be correctly calculated. Because the chipmunk, in common with all small rodents, has a small body size and high metabolic rate its potential to lose body heat and fluids during surgery is large. All small rodents are prone to hypothermia and circulatory shock when anaesthetised. These problems must be minimised by the following methods:

- The patient's body can be wrapped in aluminium foil to conserve heat.
- The shaved surgical area should be the minimum size possible, and skin preparation should be carried out using warmed preparations. Care should be taken to avoid wetting the surrounding coat as this will lead to cooling by evaporation.
- If subcutaneous fluid therapy is given the fluid must be warmed to the patient's body temperature.

ANAESTHESIA

Inhalation anaesthesia is the easiest method, using halothane, isoflurane or methoxyflurane with oxygen. For induction a small see-through chamber can be constructed to allow the anaesthetic gas to enter, with holes which permit the gas to escape and be scavenged. The patient can remain in the chamber until the righting reflex is lost and then it can be transferred to and maintained on a face mask. Small face masks can be made with the ends of plastic syringe cases. If the chipmunk has been transported in the nest box, this can be used as the induction chamber.

Halothane

Dose: The induction concentration should be 3–4%, and the maintenance concentration 1–2%.

Isoflurane

Dose: The induction concentration is 3.4–4.5%, and 1.5–3% for maintenance.

Methoxyflurane

Dose: The induction concentration is 4%, with 0.4–1% for maintenance.

Ether

Dose: Ether is not recommended because it is highly irritant and explosive.

Anaesthetic monitoring

Monitoring the anaesthetic is not as easy as in a dog or cat because the chipmunk patient is much smaller. The most reliable indicator of surgical anaesthesia is the loss of withdrawal reflex in response to a painful stimulus such as a toe, tail or ear pinch. As the anesthetic deepens the respiratory and cardiovascular parameters will be depressed.

Doxapram

Dopram (Willows Francis Ltd.)

This contains 20 mg/ml doxapram and is a useful respiratory stimulant.

Dose: 10 mg/kg can be given, i.e. 0.05 ml, by subcutaneous, intra-muscular or intraperitoneal injection.

ANALGESIA

Analgesia is most effective if given before anaesthesia, or during the anaesthetic.

Buprenorphine

Buprenorphine can be widely used.

Dose: A dose of 0.1 mg/kg can be given subcutaneously every 6–12 hours.

After surgery non-steroidal analgesics can be given by mouth.

POST-OPERATIVE CARE

The chipmunk should be kept warm and quiet. Initially the external temperature should be 35°C (95°F), reducing to 25°C (77°F) once recovery is in progress. A heat-reflective surface, e.g. Flectabed, or vetbed are suitable for this; sawdust or shavings are not recommended because they will stick to wounds and catch in the face and eyes.

Fluid-replacement therapy

This is particularly valuable following surgery, or for any debilitated chipmunks. Glucose–saline (5% glucose, 0.9% saline) is the fluid of choice.

Dose: 1–2 ml can be administered subcutaneously, or 2–3 ml via intraperitoneal injection.

DRUG TREATMENTS

Due to the nature of the patient, medication through the drinking water is the easiest method of administration. Other drugs can be mixed with a favourite food, or puréed apple. Injections are usually impossible in the conscious chipmunk.

Antibiotics

Tx 1. Enrofloxacin

Baytril (Bayer plc)

Dose: 10mg/kg daily.

The 2.5% solution can be diluted as follows: 4 ml is made up to 1 litre with water to give a concentration of 100 mg/litre.

Tx 2. Oxytetracycline

Terramycin Soluble Powder 5.5% (Pfizer Ltd.)

This contains 55 g/kg oxytetracycline hydrochloride. One level scoopful contains approximately 4 g of powder, i.e. approximately 200 mg oxytetracycline.

Dose: One level scoopful in 2 litres of drinking water gives a concentration of about 100 mg/litre; one level spoonful in 0.5 litre gives a concentration of about 400 mg/litre (equivalent to about 2 mg/5 ml).

Tx 3. Potentiated sulphonamides

Borgal 7.5% (Hoechst)

This contains 12.5 mg/ml trimethoprim and 62.5 mg/ml sulphadoxine.

Dose: 0.6 ml/kg can be given daily by subcutaneous injection (average adult dose 0.1 ml).

Tribrissen 24% injection (Mallinckrodt Veterinary Ltd.)

This contains 40 mg/ml trimethoprim and 200 mg/ml sulphadiazine.

Dose: The injection can be diluted 1–2 ml into 1 litre of water, and used as medicated drinking water.

Probiotics

These can be given at the same time as antibiotics, or in times of dehabilitation, to improve the appetite.

Tx 4. Avipro (Vetark Health)

This is a water soluble probiotic, containing *Lactobacillus acidophilus*, *Enterococcus faecium* and *Saccharomyces* with electrolytes.
   It can be diluted in the drinking water at a rate of 5 g/200 ml water.

Dose: It can be diluted in the drinking water at a rate of 5 g/200 ml water.

Comment: It is also useful in periods of stress, to protect the gastrointestinal tract from stress-related disease.

Tx 5. Enterodex (Vydex Animal Health)

This contains the beneficial bacteria *Enterococcus*, similar to *Lactobacillus*.

Dose: One teaspoonful (5 g) in the drinking water is sufficient for 40 chipmunks. For single chipmunks a small pinch can be mixed with the drinking water.

Corticosteroids

Tx 6. Dexamethasone

Dexafort (Intervet UK Ltd.)

This is a combination of long- and short-acting steroids which produces a rapid and long-lasting glucogenic effect, and a long anti-inflammatory and anti-pruritic effect.

Dose: 0.1 ml by subcutaneous or intramuscular injection.

Tx 7. Ivermectin

Ivomec Injection for Cattle (Merck, Sharpe & Dohme Ltd.)

Ivomec contains 1% w/v ivermectin.

Dose: It can be given by subcutaneous injection at a dose rate of 200–400 μg/kg every 10 days. The cattle injection can be diluted 1:10 with water and 0.02 ml given by injection.

Alternatively undiluted Ivomec can be given by mouth at a dose of 1 drop, repeated at 10 day intervals as necessary.

Tx 8. Calcium supplementation

Callo-Cal D (C-Vet)

This contains 0.75% w/v colloidal calcium oleate and 70 i.u./ml vitamin D.

Dose: 0.1 ml may be given orally daily.

Tx 9. Cloxacillin

Orbenin Ophthalmic Ointment (Pfizer Ltd.)

This contains 500 mg cloxacillin in 3 g of suspension.

Dose: Apply once daily.

Tx 10. Fipronil

Frontline (Rhône Mérieux)

This contains 0.25% w/v fipronil.

Dose: 7.5 mg/kg may be given. It may be necessary to dilute with iso-propyl alcohol to achieve a dose of 7.5 mg/kg, and used as a spray.

GERBILS

Gerbils are one of the most recent small pets, having first been introduced into Britain in 1964. Although there are about 80 species in the wild, the species most usually kept as a pet is the Mongolian gerbil (*Meriones unguiculatus*) also referred to as the clawed jird by zoologists. This species is native to the desert and semi-desert areas of Mongolia and north-eastern China.

Shaw's jird (*Meriones shawii*) is in the same family as the Mongolian gerbil and although once a laboratory animal is now also being kept as a pet. It is larger than the Mongolian gerbil, but possesses many similar characteristics. Shaw's jird originates from the dry areas of north Africa and the Middle East, living in deep burrows in the sand.

The gerbil's body is specifically adapted for its natural desert habitat. Gerbils are able to conserve liquid, and produce small amounts of a highly concentrated urine and dry faeces. They therefore make very clean pets with no smell.

Generally, gerbils are infrequently affected by disease; however, their housing and environment can have dramatic effects on their health, and the majority of their diseases are stress-related.

Gerbils are diurnal, and are active both day and night.

7 HUSBANDRY AND NUTRITION

Housing

Mongolian gerbils

In the natural state gerbils live in deep complex burrows in sandy soils. They are social animals and are happiest kept in groups. The most natural form of accommodation in captivity is the gerbilarium, a glass or plastic aquarium covered with wire mesh to prevent escape and with deep burrowing medium. Wire or plastic cages can also be used. Wooden cages are unsuitable as they are likely to be gnawed. If a cage is used a nest box should be provided to offer some privacy if the gerbils are unable to burrow.

The minimum cage size for two Mongolian gerbils is 60 cm × 25 cm × 25 cm (l × w × h). However, the larger the cage the better, because a large cage will encourage exercise and prevent boredom. As a guide 750 cm^2 should be allowed per gerbil. If an exercise wheel is provided it must be a solid type, as gerbils can trap their legs and tails in open wire wheels. The wheels are best left in for only part of a day because overuse can lead to exhaustion.

Bedding: In the gerbilarium the preferred burrowing medium is a layer of moss peat and chopped straw at least 10 cm deep. Shredded white paper is suitable for bedding, but synthetic bedding should be avoided because it may cause stomach impaction if ingested. Synethetic fibres can also become wrapped around limbs and toes, causing serious damage. Shredded paper or newspaper with ink should be avoided because the ink may be poisonous.

Alternatively, cage floors can be covered with sawdust or wood shavings. Although sawdust is more absorbent it easily clings to the fur and fresh foods and may cause eye irritation. If either sawdust or wood shavings are used as floor litter it is important that they are made only from untreated soft woods, as certain hard woods have toxic properties.

Sand is rarely used as it may stain the fur, and like sawdust, cause eye irritation. However, a small quantity of fine sand can be provided in a dish for a sand bath.

Meadow hay makes an excellent bedding material, but care must be taken to make sure it stays dry and does not become mouldy.

Shaw's jirds

The requirements of Shaw's jirds are similar to those of the Mongolian gerbil, with a little more space. Large aquariums can be used, with a base of wood chippings. Pipes and jars can be buried under the surface to create an environment similar to their natural habitat.

Environment

A gerbilarium must not be sited near a radiator or in direct sunlight because overheating of the tank can lead to heat exhaustion. The room temperature should be between 15 and 20°C (59–68°F). Gerbils are diurnal; they are active during the day and need playthings such as cardboard tubes to prevent boredom. Metal, plastic and painted wooden toys should be avoided as should objects made of foam or fabric which could be ingested.

In good weather gerbils can be allowed to exercise outside in small mesh runs with solid bottoms, providing they are protected from predators. Wire mesh floors should not be used as these may predispose to sore hocks.

Stocking

Mongolian gerbils

Mongolian gerbils are social animals and prefer to be kept in groups. Groups of females will live in harmony. Males can coexist, but only if introduced to each other at an early age, or ideally from the same litter and even then they may begin fighting. The more space that is available for the group of gerbils, the less likely they are to fight.

If breeding, Mongolian gerbils can be kept as monogamous pairs, or as harems, with one male and several females. Any pairing should be done before 10 weeks of age to prevent fighting. If introducing a female to a male after this age, she should be introduced into his environment and not vice versa. In a monogamous pair the male will help bring up the offspring and can be safely left with the female and her litter.

Shaw's jirds

Males can be kept as pairs, especially if they are introduced young, or are from the same litter. Female Shaw's jirds tend to be very territorial and dominant; they can be aggressive, and are best kept singly. Two females from the same litter may live together, although they are likely to start fighting once they reach maturity.

Hygiene

As the gerbil is adapted for desert life and produces little waste it is a very clean animal. In a gerbilarium with absorbent burrowing medium and bedding the gerbils can live for up to 3 months in sanitary conditions before requiring a change, and this makes them ideal pets for the classroom.

If floor litter is used in a cage it will need to be changed weekly, but the nest box need not be disturbed. It is important to check the cage daily and remove any stale or mouldy food before it gets buried.

Nutrition

Mongolian gerbils

In the wild the Mongolian gerbil's diet consists of seeds, grains, roots, leaves and stems. Proprietary gerbil mixes containing sunflower seeds, wheat, maize, millet, oats and barley imitate this diet. The mix should be fed once a day, and any surplus removed so that it is not allowed to become stale. An adult gerbil will consume approximately 15 g/day. The mixed seed diet should be supplemented with fresh fruit and vegetables such as banana, apple, carrot, lettuce, etc. Extra protein can be given in the form of hard-boiled eggs, cheese, and milk powder. Animal proteins such as meat, cat and dog food can be given in small quantities. Extra carbohydrates such as baked bread and dog biscuits can be given, and these are useful to satisfy the gnawing requirements. All fresh food must be washed because gerbiils are very susceptible to insecticide residues on vegetables.

Any new food must be introduced gradually in small quantities to avoid causing diarrhoea. As with other rodents, gerbils may selectively eat sunflower seeds which have a low calcium content and are high in fat. An excess of these can cause calcium deficiency, fractures and obesity. Gerbils which eat too much fat readily develop lipaemia and hepatic lipidosis. For this reason sunflower seeds should make up less than 10% of the daily ration. If peanuts are fed they must be of good quality; mouldy peanuts may contain aflatoxins which will cause fatal liver damage. A variety of wild plants can also be fed, e.g. dandelion, shepherd's purse, groundsel, chickweed and plantain.

Despite their adaptation to desert life, gerbils require a regular supply of water. Lack of water can lead to infertility. Water should be provided from a dropper bottle, but gerbils drink very little (an adult gerbil will drink between 4 and 10 ml/day), and if fed greens they may drink nothing at all.

Pregnant and lactating gerbils can be given extra protein such as cheese and egg. Powdered milk can also be offered sprinkled on fruit. Fresh water must be available because their water requirement increases. Vitamin drops formulated for gerbils can also be given.

Young gerbils will start eating solid food at 2–3 weeks of age and should be weaned by 4 weeks of age. Their first solid food should be small seeds (canary rearing seed) and a little washed fruit and vegetables. Proteins such as egg and cheese should not be introduced until they are 6 weeks old. Eating habits are acquired at an early age, so it is important that a variety of foodstuffs are offered early on to prevent the development of finicky eating. Fresh water must be available; it is important that water bottles are at a height which is within reach of the young gerbils.

Shaw's jirds

The diet of the Shaw's jird is similar to that of the Mongolain gerbil, a seed mix supplemented with fruit and vegetables. Shaw's jirds can also be given meat proteins; either cat or dog food, or mealworms are suitable.

8 SYSTEMS AND DISEASES

THE SKIN

Gerbils secrete an oil with which they groom their coats, and in their natural environment this oil evaporates. If the humidity in captivity is too high this oil will remain on the coat giving a greasy appearance. The recommended relative humidity is 45–55%. Above 55% relative humidity the coat will also appear roughened.

A rough coat may also be a non-specific sign of disease, malnutrition or stress.

Sebaceous gland

This gland is present on the mid-ventral abdomen and it produces a yellow-brown secretion used for scent marking. It is under androgen control and is twice as large in the male as the female. The sebaceons gland may become infected and inflamed, it may also turn neoplastic in the older gerbil, both adenomas and carcinomas having been recorded.

Treatment: Topical therapy for infection. Surgical resection of tumours can be attempted, although haemorrhage from the site is common. Hormonal therapy with megestrol acetate (Tx 20. Ovarid) at a dose of 1 mg on alternate days has been reported to have been used to decrease the activity of this gland (R.S. Proverbs, personal communication).

Barbering

Clinical signs: There may be hair loss, or areas where the hair is chewed short, particularly around the tail base. It may be due to the gerbil chewing its own fur, or being chewed by another member of the group. Gerbils may also rub themselves on their cage equipment and cause hair loss.

Treatment and prevention: Barbering occurs due to stress, overcrowding and boredom. These factors should be corrected; more playthings can be introduced, and also some bedding such as meadow hay could be added.

Nasal alopecia

Clinical signs: Hair loss on the nose. This occurs as some gerbils persistently rub their noses on the cage bars.

Treatment and prevention: If secondary infection is present topical antibiotics (Tx 6. Chlortetracycline ointment) should be used. The gerbil should be transferred from a cage to an aquarium type enclosure and the hair should regrow.

Sore nose

This is also referred to as facial dermatitis: see Respiratory System.

Staphylococcal dermatitis

Clinical signs: There are inflamed areas of skin which may become ulcerated. These areas may develop from bite wounds, or the bacteria may enter through small abrasions caused by burrowing in rough bedding. Infection by *Staphylococcus* species is also a common sequel in nasal dermatitis.

Staphylococcus aureus is associated with an endemic dermatitis in young gerbils of weaning age, and mortality may be as high as 25%.

Treatment: Antibiotics (Tx 1–5) may be given orally and topically. Abrasive bedding should be removed and, if fighting is the causal factor, stress and overcrowding should be reduced.

Ectoparasites

Demodecosis

Clinical signs: The disease may start as small blisters on the skin of the hindquarters, feet or ears. These blisters then erupt and the fur is lost. The skin is dry, flaky and inflamed. It is generally seen only if the gerbil is debilitated (e.g. old, pregnant, malnourished, under stress). The causal agent is *Demodex merioni*.

Treatment: Mange dressing, e.g. amitraz (Tx 12. Aludex). It may require 3–6 treatments at fortnightly intervals. Ivermectin (Tx. 13) can be given by mouth. Stress factors must be eliminated. The affected animal should be isolated. Vitamin supplements are useful, or the gerbil can be given pieces of fresh orange or small vitamin C tablets to chew.

Other external parasites (fleas, lice) are not common in gerbils, and only result from contact with other animals. If the gerbils are housed in old bird cages it is possible for them to acquire red mites. These cause pruritus, and also an anaemia which may be fatal in young gerbils.

Ringworm

Clinical signs: Alopecia and hyperkeratosis occur. The causal agents are *Trichophyton mentagrophytes* and *Microsporum gypseum*.

Diagnosis: Microscopy and culture on Sabouraud's medium are required.

Treatment: Griseofulvin (Tx 9) should be given at a dose of 25 mg/kg twice daily for at least a month. This approximates to a dose of 2.5 mg twice daily for an adult gerbil. Shampooing with a povidone–iodine solution (Tx 10) or 4% chlorhexidine (Tx 11. *Hibbiscrub*) is also recommended. The cage should also be thoroughly cleaned with the povidone-iodine solution (Tx 10) and the bedding changed.

Comment: As ringworm is a zoonosis the animal should be handled only with gloves for treatment.

Cutaneous neoplasms

Squamous cell carcinomas and melanomas have been recorded in gerbils.

THE REPRODUCTIVE SYSTEM

Litter size: 4–6
Birth weight: 2.5–3.5 g
Weaning age: 21–28 days
Eyes open: 10–12 days
Weaning weight: 11-18 g
Puberty: males 10–12 weeks
          females 12–14 weeks
Best age to breed: males 5 months
                females 3–4 months
Retire from breeding: males 2 years
              females 18 months
Oestrus: every 6 days throughout the year
Post-partum oestrus: fertile
Duration of oestrus: 12–18 hours; mating generally takes place at night
Gestation: 24–26 days
The female gerbil has four pairs of teats, two thoracic and two inguinal.

Sexing

The anogenital distance in the male is twice that of the female. In an adult male this distance is 10 mm, compared with 5 mm in the adult female (Figure 8.1). Sexing should be possible from the age of 4 weeks. At this age the scrotal sacs of the male will also become evident.

The mid-ventral scent gland is androgen sensitive and therefore twice as large in the male than the female.

Breeding

Mongolian gerbils

Many sources suggest that Mongolian gerbils form monogamous pairs and pair for life; however, this is not always the case. They are best introduced at 8–10 weeks of age (i.e. before sexual maturity) to prevent fighting. If gerbils are to be paired purely for mating they must be introduced in a neutral cage, or the female introduced to the male, and never vice versa or they will fight.

Oestrus occurs every 6 days throughout the year, and lasts overnight.

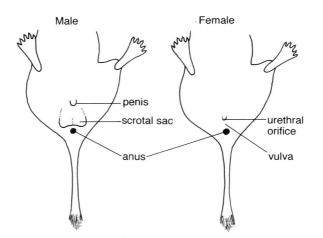

Figure 8.1 External genitalia.

During oestrus the mating process may go on for several hours over which time there may be several hundred mountings. The female does not produce a visible copulatory plug in the vent (unlike chinchillas and mice) but there is generally a sore evident in this area in both male and female which will heal in 2–3 days.

Mongolian gerbils also exhibit a post-partum oestrus, which lasts for about 5 hours after the birth, and they can rebreed after parturition. If mated at the post-partum oestrus delayed implantation may occur if the gerbil is suckling more than two young. Implantation can be delayed for up to 2 weeks, so gestation can be as long as 48 days. Gerbils do not mate whilst lactating, and exhibit their next oestrus post-weaning.

Shaw's jirds

Female Shaw's jirds will only accept the male when they are in season, and even then the female may only tolerate the male in her cage for 1–2 hours. If the male is placed where the pair can smell each other the female will wag her tail vigorously if she is in season. If she is not, she will squeak and attempt to attack the male.

There is a fertile post-partum oestrus, but any litters born as a result of mating at this time are likely to be neglected.

The young are born blind and naked, but develop quickly, and by 16 days of age are mobile, fully furred and eating some solid food.

Pseudopregnancy

If there is a sterile mating the female may exhibit pseudopregnancy. This lasts 14–16 days.

Gestation

During pregnancy the female should not be handled unless it is essential. She should be supplied with plenty of nesting material, and given calcium- and protein-rich foods, such as eggs and powdered milk in small quantities. Sunflower seeds should be rationed to prevent unnecessary obesity which may lead to dystocia.

Parturition

Parturition generally occurs at night. The young gerbils are born blind, naked and helpless. They should be left in the nest undisturbed. Both the male and female take care of the offspring and by 7 days of age they have a thin covering of fur. The eyes of the young start to open at 10 days of age and their incisors erupt at 12–14 days.

Some breeders prefer to remove the male before parturition to prevent rebreeding at the post-partum oestrus. He should not be kept away for more than 2 weeks as the pair may fight when reintroduced.

Problems after parturition

Cannibalism

Rarely, a female will kill and cannibalise all or part of her litter. This may be due to agalactia, mastitis, or her inborn instinct to recognise an abnormal youngster. The young may also be abandoned if there is too little nesting material, or not enough privacy for the nest box. Cannibalism may also occur if the female is disturbed. It is thought that in some cases cannibalism may be an inherited behavioural trait. One of the commonest causes of cannibalism is lack of food or water.

Fostering

Fostering may be necessary if the female dies after parturition, or produces an exceptionally large litter. If more than one female is kept in the breeding pen with the male then another female can take over the task of rearing the young. If the baby gerbils from a large litter are to be fostered out they should be removed when both the male and female are away from the nest. The baby gerbils should be rubbed with some urine stained bedding of the foster parents so that they pick up this scent and are less likely to be rejected. Alternatively the babies can be covered with wheatgerm, which will encourage the foster mother to clean them and as she does so she will cover them with her scent. Hand feeding is difficult.

Weaning

Weaning is normally completed around 21 days of age. The young gerbils should initially be offered soft mashes with seeds and bread soaked in milk. Their first solid food should be small seeds and a little soft fruit and vegetables. Both food and water must be offered, and be accessible from 14 days. Water bottles must be placed within reach of the young gerbils. If food and water are denied from days 16–25, infant mortality is high. Proteins such as eggs and cheese should not be introduced until 6 weeks of age.

Infertility

- *Poor husbandry and nutrition* may result in failure to breed.
- *Inadequate water supply* may lead to infertility.
- As the gerbils form monogamous pairs, the death or removal of one or other partner may lead to the infertility or pregnancy failure of the remaining partner.
- An overfat female may be infertile; she should be put on a calorie-reduced diet and encouraged to exercise.
- Environmental factors. The mating cage should be clean and well ventilated. A 12 hour daylight/12 hour darkness lighting system is necessary for optimum breeding potential. The cage must offer space, nesting material and privacy. An absence of any of these factors may result in infertility. Gerbils may also fail to breed if they can smell other predators such as rats, cats or dogs. Chemical and disinfectant smells may also discourage breeding.
- *Ovarian and uterine tumours*. These are the commonest reported neoplasms in gerbils, and cystic ovaries are very common in older females. Females stop ovulating and cease to breed at around 2 years of

age. As females reach this age their litters are likely to be smaller and less vigorous.

- *Ovarian cysts.* These are common in the older female, and a cause of infertility. The cysts can reach such a size that the gerbil looks full term pregnant. Large cysts cause abdominal discomfort, inappetance and lethargy. Treatment is by ovariohysterectomy.

THE URINARY SYSTEM

Polydipsia and subsequent polyuria are a finding in the older gerbil. The two common causes are diabetes, and chronic interstitial nephritis.

Diabetes is secondary to overactive adrenal glands causing hyperlipidaemia and hyperglycaemia, and obese animals are most prone to developing the condition. Chronic interstitial nephritis is characterised by polydipsia and weight loss, and a raised blood–urea nitrogen (the normal level is 20 mg/dl and a raised level is 30 mg/dl). Affected gerbils can be supported with vitamin supplementation and fluid administration, e.g. Tx 18. Lectade.

THE RESPIRATORY SYSTEM

Respiratory infections

Clinical signs: Upper respiratory tract infections, with symptoms of sneezing and coryza can be caught from humans with colds, and are common in school gerbils. The bacteria which are responsible for such cross infection are ß-haemolytic streptococci. Infection will spread between in-contact gerbils.

Treatment: The affected gerbil should be isolated and kept warm. Mild cases will resolve in 2–3 days. Antibiotic eye cream can be applied, and antibiotics administered in the drinking water (Tx 1–5). A little mentholated ointment (e.g. Vick) can be rubbed on the inside of the cage to help clear the nasal passages. The feeding of a little oily fish is said to lubricate the nasal passages.

Comment: Similar symptoms will occur if the bedding is an irritant, e.g. sawdust. Abrasive bedding, e.g. sand, may cause small abrasions via which *Streptococcus* spp. may enter and cause infection. Other predisposing factors are draughts and the build up of ammonia from soiled bedding, and these should be avoided.

Sore nose (nasal dermatitis)

Clinical signs: A sore nose and sore eyes, often associated with bleeding and ulceration, are seen. Nasal dermatitis may result from the gerbils' habit of burrowing and causing small facial abrasions. It is commonly associated with an excessive accumulation of porphyrins around the nasal area. These porphyrins are produced by the Harderian glands in the eye and are usually removed continuously as the gerbil grooms itself with its forepaws (they are responsible for the red colouration of the tears). If the porphyrins are allowed to accumulate they are highly irritant. Often *Staphylococcus* spp. are identified associated with the dermatitis.

Treatment: The nose can be regularly cleaned with a mild saline solution (1 teaspoon of salt to 1 pint of water or 5 g salt to 500 ml of water). Removing any stress factors (e.g. by introducing a compatible cage mate, increasing the environmental space, or reducing overcrowding) may reduce porphyrin secretion. More absorbent bedding may help to clean the gerbil's face as it burrows. Surgical resection of the Harderian glands will produce a cure in chronic cases.

   Where secondary infection is present this may be treated with topical or oral antibiotics (Tx 1–5). Chloramphenicol or tetracycline preparations (Tx 2 and 3) are the most effective. Associated conjunctivitis can be treated with eye ointments (Tx 21 and 22).

Comment: Stress factors must be eliminated as they are a double trigger in the development of nasal dermatitis. Environmental stresses of overcrowding and high humidity are particularly associated with this condition. Stressed gerbils will spend more time burrowing and are more likely to develop facial abrasions. Stress also leads to increased porphyrin secretion by the Harderian glands.

THE EYE

Gerbils will often produce red (porphyrin containing) tears associated with stress. If these build up they become highly irritant and lead to nasal dermatitis.

Conjunctivitis

Clinical signs: These include excessive lacrimation and inflamed conjunctiva.

Treatment: Antibiotic/steroid eye cream, or drops (Tx 22. Neobiotic HC).

Excess dust, an allergy to the bedding material, and abrasive bedding can all cause excessive lacrimation, and abrasive bedding can also cause corneal ulceration. These factors should all be considered when treating conjunctivitis.

THE EAR

Ear infections

Clinical signs: Torticollis, circling and loss of balance. Infection of the middle and inner ear may follow respiratory infections, or may be the only presenting sign of infection.

Treatment: Antibiotics (Tx 1–5) and corticosteroids (Tx 16) may be used.

Comment: Gerbils appear to have a resistance to otitis media, and it is seen infrequently. The gerbil has good ear drainage compared with other rodents.

Aural neoplasia

Clinical signs: There is a keratinized mass in the external ear which may extend to the middle ear. There may be a head tilt, or hair loss around the ears. The growth is an aural cholesteatoma, and is most commonly seen in gerbils over the age of 2 years.

THE DIGESTIVE SYSTEM

Coprophagy

Coprophagy is a normal process; however, it may only be seen to occur if the gerbil is not on a balanced diet. Well fed gerbils may not always be coprophagic.

Malocclusion

As with all rodents, the gerbil's teeth are open rooted and grow throughout life. It is essential that they are provided with adequate food and toys to gnaw. Occasionally the incisors are not aligned properly and are not worn down by gnawing.

Treatment: The teeth can be clipped as regularly as necessary. Affected individuals should not be bred from. Incisor overgrowth can be curbed by the provision of wholemeal macaroni, apple twigs, gerbil chews, nuts or dog biscuits to gnaw.

Diarrhoea

This may be due to a dietary disturbance or, more seriously, infectious disease.

Diet induced diarrhoea

A dramatic dietary change or the consumption of stale food will lead to scouring.

Clinical signs: The affected animal holds a 'tucked-up' posture, huddled in a corner, with faecal soiling around the anus.

Treatment: If the diarrhoea is associated with dietary change all foodstuffs should be removed. A kaolin/pectin (Tx 17) mixture can be given or, more traditionally, arrowroot powder or arrowroot biscuits can be used for their astringent properties. Raspberry leaves, burnt toast and apple peel are also all astringent and can be given too. Good quality hay can be introduced first, followed by the dry mix. Fluid intake is important; if necessary fluid therapy can be administered, or fluid replacement (e.g. Tx 18. Lectade) given by mouth. If only one gerbil is affected it may be better not to separate it from its pair, as this would cause extra stress.

   If the gerbil is anorexic it can be tempted with dehusked sunflower seeds to encourage it to eat. Probiotics (e.g. Tx 7. Avipro) can also help to stimulate the appetite.

Colibacillosis

Diarrhoea in young gerbils of 10 days old to weaning may be caused by *Escherichia coli* and be associated with stress.

Treatment: Provision of warmth, with administration of antibiotics (Tx 4. Neobiotic) and a kaolin/pectin mixture (Tx 17) is necessary. Corticosteroids (Tx 16) can also be given. A probiotic (Tx 7. Avipro) may also aid recovery. Prevention should be aimed at removing any stress factors and improving hygiene.

Salmonellosis

Diarrhoea caused by *Salmonella* is uncommon, but infection can be contracted if the food is contaminated by mice carrying *Salmonella typhimurium*. There is no carrier state in gerbils, and affected individuals usually recover from the disease. Occasionally it may cause septicaemia. Care should be taken as it is a zoonosis.

Clinical signs: These include dehydration, rough coat, abdominal bloat with diarrhoea. In the males the testes may be swollen.

Diagnosis: Culture of the blood or faeces.

Tyzzer's disease

This is caused by infection with the bacterium *Bacillus piliformis*. The most common form of infection is sub-clinical with a persistence of carriers, and outbreaks of disease are seen associated with stress. The most commonly affected groups are weanling gerbils and nursing females.

Tyzzer's disease is usually introduced by carrier rodents which contaminate food and bedding. It is spread by the faecal–oral route and it can survive for periods over a year in its spore form in bedding or feed.

Clinical signs: The acute form in weanling or stressed animals will cause lethargy, anorexia, rough hair coat and death within 48–72 hours. A watery diarrhoea is common, but not always seen. The chronic form reflects the hepatic lesions which occur, and affected individuals exhibit weight loss, rough hair coat and death. If the central nervous system is affected individuals will show torticollis, loss of balance and death.

Diagnosis: At post-mortem the most consistent change is an enlarged liver which contains numerous white, yellow or grey necrotic foci. In the intestines there may be oedema and haemorrhage around the ileocaecal-colic junction.

Giemsa stains of hepatocytes will exhibit the filamentous Gram–negative organism.

Treatment: Treatment of the acute form is difficult. Antibiotic therapy with oxytetracycline or neomycin (Tx 3 and 4) can be tried to control the diarrhoea, together with supportive measures such as warmth, fluids and vitamins. Oxytetracycline in the drinking water at a rate of 100 mg/litre can be used to suppress an outbreak amongst in-contact stock. Oxytetracycline (Tx 3) is the drug of choice because it is not absorbed from the gut and produces therapeutic levels in the intestine whilst maintaining low serum concentration.

Prevention: Hygiene and protection from contamination by rodents is important. Although antibiotics may suppress an outbreak they may induce the carrier state and disease will reoccur if the carrier animals are stressed.

The bacterium can survive as spores which are resistant to ethanol and quaternary ammonium compounds; however, a 0.5% sodium hypochlorite solution and peracetic acid will inactivate the spores.

Constipation

Clinical signs: An absence of droppings, or scant amount of faeces and abdominal discomfort may be evident. The abdomen may appear bloated. Similar signs will also be seen with impaction, usually caused by ingestion of unsuitable bedding material.

Treatment: Provision of green food is beneficial; if available, dandelion leaves have a laxative effect. If constipation is accompanied by bloating two or three drops of cod-liver oil can be given orally. Where intestinal impaction is suspected cod-liver oil or a few drops of liquid paraffin can be given by mouth in an attempt to shift the obstruction.

Endoparasites

Gerbils can carry *Hymenolepis nana* and *Taenia crassicollis*.

Clinical signs: Infection may be sub-clinical unless the host is debilitated, and in the latter these parasites may cause enteritis and weight loss. *Hymenolepis nana* is zoonotic.

Diagnosis: Faecal examination will reveal the hook-like ova of *Hymenolepis nana*. Adult tapeworms live in the small intestine and may be found in the pancreatic and bile ducts.

Treatment: Niclosamide (Tx 15. Troscan 100) can be given at a dose of 100 mg/kg and repeated after 7 days. Troscan 100 contains 100 mg niclosamide and one tenth of a tablet can be crushed and administered orally.

Comment: Gerbils can also carry pinworms *Denstomella translucida* in their small intestine and a mouse/rat pinworm in their large intestine. These can be treated with Ivermectin (Tx 13), given orally or by injection.

THE MUSCULOSKELETAL SYSTEM

Fractures

Trauma such as a fall may result in a limb fracture. If the gerbil's diet is made up of more than 10% sunflower seeds it may have sub-clinical calcium deficiency and be more prone to spontaneous fractures. Distal limb fractures may heal with a light supportive dressing for 10–14 days. Fracture healing occurs rapidly with a callus forming in the first 7–10 days. More severe comminuted fractures may require limb amputation.

BEHAVIOUR AND THE CENTRAL NERVOUS SYSTEM

Foot stamping

Gerbils will drum their feet as a sign of territorial warning. They foot stamp in the presence of a female in season and will also exhibit displeasure in this way.

Aggression

Mongolian gerbils

Gerbils form monogamous pairs and any alteration or change in the social structure may lead to fighting. Gerbils are best paired before sexual maturity (10 weeks). Pairs formed after this time may become aggressive. If pairing sexually mature males and females they should be introduced on neutral territory. Fighting is most likely to occur if the female is not in season. If fighting does occur it is best to separate them and try again in 4–5 days when the female may be on heat. It may be preferable to put them in a cage with a mesh partition which can be removed once they accept each other. If no neutral cage is available the female should always be introduced onto the male's territory and not vice versa.

Overcrowding or malnutrition will also lead to aggression. Gerbils will fight to the death and it is important to separate them quickly if necessary. It may be possible to facilitate the introduction of two gerbils by dusting them with talcum powde., to mask their individual scents and make acceptance more likely.

Shaw's jirds

See Chapter 7, Stocking.

Epilepsy

Epileptiform seizures may be initiated by stress, handling, environmental change and anaesthesia, and may occur in as much as 20% of the population. They usually develop after 2 months of age, with a peak of severity at 6 months. Epilepsy is thought to be an inherited trait in some strains. There appears to be no long-lasting effect from the seizures, and it is suggested that they are a protective device in the wild to deter predators.

If treatment is necessary anti-epileptic drugs, e.g. primidone (Tx 19. Mysoline) can be used; however these drugs may prove toxic. If possible gerbils that exhibit this trait should be removed from the breeding programme.

MISCELLANEOUS CONDITIONS

Heat stroke

Although the gerbil is a desert animal in its natural environment, it is able to survive the heat of the desert by deep burrowing in the sand. Such behaviour is not generally possible in captivity and the gerbil will become uncomfortable above 35°C (95°F). Heat tolerance will also decrease as humidity increases.

Clinical signs: Collapse, panting and trembling may be observed.

Treatment: The gerbil should be moved to a cooler, well-ventilated room. The gerbil can be wrapped in a cloth soaked in cool water. Fluids can be administered by mouth.

9 ANAESTHESIA AND DRUG TREATMENTS

HANDLING

Gerbils are best supported cupped in the palm of the hand and steadied by holding the base of the tail. They can also be restrained by the scruff. They should never be picked up by the tail itself as it may deglove and slough off. Injuries to the tail are complicated by haemorrhage which must be stopped using a styptic such as potash alum or a styptic pencil. If the whole tail is shed the stump should heal.

NURSING

The general principles of nursing are to provide a warm and stress-free environment. Depending upon the condition of the patient it may be preferable to keep it with its mate because the stress of separation may lead to further stress and depression. In the home warmth is easily provided by the airing cupboard.

PRE-ANAESTHETIC PREPARATION

Pre-anaesthetic starvation is unnecessary because regurgitation cannot occur due to the anatomy of the cardia of the stomach. Water should also remain available as any restriction can exaggerate the metabolic effects of anaesthesia.

The patient must be accurately weighed to enable drug doses to be correctly calculated. Because the gerbil, in common with all small rodents has a small body size and high metabolic rate its potential to lose body heat and fluids during surgery is large. All small rodents are prone to hypothermia and circulatory shock when anaesthetised. These problems must be minimised by the following methods:

- The patient's body can be wrapped in aluminium foil to conserve heat.
- The shaved surgical area should be the minimum size possible, and skin preparation should be carried out using warmed preparations. Care should be taken to avoid wetting the surrounding coat as this will lead to cooling by evaporation.
- If subcutaneous fluid therapy is given the fluid must be warmed to the patient's body temperature.

PREMEDICATION

Atropine should be given as a premedicant at a dose of 40 µg/kg by either subcutaneous or intramuscular injection to reduce salivation.

Dose: Atropine sulphate injection contains 600 µg/ml. An adult gerbil weighing 100 g requires a dose of of 0.006 ml subcutaneously. The atropine sulphate injection can be diluted 1:10 with sterile water for injection, providing a dose size of 0.06 ml.

ANAESTHESIA

Inhalation anaesthesia

Inhalation anaesthesia is the easiest method using halothane, isoflurane or methoxyflurane with an oxygen/nitrous oxide combination. For induction a small see-through chamber can be constructed to allow the anaesthetic gas to enter, with holes which permit the gas to escape and be scavenged. The patient can remain in the chamber until the righting reflex is lost and then it can be transferred to and maintained on a face mask. Small face masks can be made with the ends of plastic syringe cases.

Halothane

Dose: The induction concentration should be 3–4%, and the maintenance concentration 1–2%.

Isoflurane

Dose: The induction concentration is 3.4–4.5%, and 1.5–3% is needed for maintenance.

Methoxyflurane

Dose: The induction concentration is 4%, with 0.4–1% for maintenance.

Ether

Ether is not recommended because it is highly irritant and explosive.

Injection anaesthesia

Injectable anaesthetics are available, and can be used. The size of the patient dictates that the injections are given subcutaneously, intramuscularly or intraperitoneally. Accurate dosing is essential.

Ketamine/acepromazine and ketamine/xylazine are readily available combinations; both can be given by intraperitoneal injection.

Ketamine/acepromazine

Dose: 75 mg/kg ketamine and 3 mg/kg acepromazine intraperitoneally.

Ketamine/xylazine

Dose: 50 mg/kg ketamine and 2 mg/kg xylazine intraperitoneally.

Comment: Even when an injectable anaesthetic is used, it is recommended that oxygen should be administered through the face mask during the operative procedure.

Anaesthetic monitoring

Monitoring the anaesthetic is not as easy as in a dog or cat because the gerbil patient is much smaller. The most reliable indicator of surgical anaesthesia is the loss of withdrawal reflex in response to a painful stimulus such as a toe, tail or ear pinch. As the anaesthetic deepens the respiratory and cardiovascular parameters will be depressed.

Doxapram

Dopram (Willows Francis Ltd.)

This contains 20 mg/ml doxapram and is a useful respiratory stimulant.

Dose: 10 mg/kg can be given by subcutaneous or intramuscular injection.

ANALGESIA

Analgesia is most effective if given before anaesthesia, or during the anaesthetic.

Buprenorphine

Buprenorphine is widely used.

Dose: A dose of 0.1 mg/kg can be given subcutaneously every 6–12 hours.

After surgery non-steroidal analgesics can be given by mouth.

POST-OPERATIVE CARE

The gerbil should be kept warm and quiet. Initially the external temperature should be 35°C (95°F), reducing to 25°C (77°F) once recovery is in progress. A heat-reflective surface, e.g. Flectabed, or vetbed is suitable; sawdust or shavings are not recommended as bedding because they will stick to wounds, and catch in the face and eyes.

Fluid replacement therapy

This is particularly valuable following surgery, or for any debilitated gerbil.

Dose: Dextrose–saline (0.9% saline, 5% glucose) is the fluid of choice. 1–2 ml can be administered subcutaneously, or 2–3 ml via intraperitoneal injection.

INJECTION PROCEDURES

Subcutaneous injections can be made in the scruff of the neck, and up to 2–3 ml can be given via this route, using a 23–25 gauge needle.

Intramuscular injections can be given into the gluteal muscle using a 25 gauge needle. The maximum volume that can be given in this site is 0.05 ml.

Intraperitoneal injections can be made with a 25 gauge needle. The gerbil should be held on its back with one hind leg extended. The needle can be introduced along the line of this leg into the centre of the corresponding posterior quadrant of the abdomen. 1–2 ml can be given by this route.

Intravenous injections are very difficult due to the small size of the patient, the lateral tail vein is used for this procedure.

DRUG TREATMENTS

Because of their small size injections are best given by the subcutaneous, intraperitoneal or intramuscular routes (very small quantities only). Because of the small doses involved it is recommended that an insulin syringe be used for greatest accuracy. Drugs can also be given orally directly. If medicating the water it must be realised that the healthy gerbil drinks very little, and the sick gerbil may drink less. Water medication must be palatable, and to achieve this blackcurrant syrup (Ribena, Smith Kline Beecham) can be added to the water.

As with all small rodents gerbils have a high metabolic rate which may mean that higher dose rates are needed, and dosing may be required frequently.

Antibiotics

In common with other rodents only broad spectrum antibiotics should be used. Narrow spectrum antibiotics, with an activity against Gram-positive bacteria allow the overgrowth of *Clostridium* spp., especially *Clostridium difficile*, and a resultant fatal enterotoxaemia.

Both B vitamins and a probiotic (Tx 6) should be administered concurrently with antibiotics.

Tx 1. Enrofloxacin

Baytril (Bayer plc)

Dose: 10mg/kg daily.
The 2.5% injection solution can be given subcutaneously at a dose of 0.02 ml/day. The 2.5% oral solution can be diluted 1:1 with blackcurrant syrup and given from a dropper bottle at a dose of 1 drop twice daily.

Drinking water can be medicated with the 2.5% oral solution diluted to produce a concentration of 100 mg/litre. This can be achieved by taking 4 ml of the 2.5% oral solution and making it up to 1 litre with water.

Tx 2. Chloramphenicol

Chloramphenicol Injectable Suspension (Willows Francis)

This contains 150 mg/ml chloramphenicol PhEur.

Dose: 30 mg/kg can be given by subcutaneous injection. This approximates to a dose of 0.02 ml daily.

Tx 3. Oxytetracycline

Terramycin Soluble Powder 5.5% (Pfizer Ltd.)

Engemycin Injection 5% (Mycofarm Ltd.)

Oxytetracycline is the antibiotic of choice for Tyzzer's disease.

Dose: 20 mg/kg may be given by subcutaneous injection for 5–7 days. Tetracyclines are poorly absorbed when given orally and high oral concentrations will only produce low serum concentrations. However, water can be medicated at a concentration of 100 mg/litre. When using the 5.5% soluble powder this is equivalent to one level scoopful (approximately 4 g) dissolved in 2 litres of water (one level scoopful weighs 4 g and contains approximately 200 mg oxytetracycline).

Tx 4. Neomycin

Neobiotic Aquadrops (Upjohn Ltd.)

These contain 50 mg/ml neomycin sulphate. Upon dosing orally, 90% of the neomycin remains in the gut, and little is absorbed systemically.

Dose: The aquadrops can be diluted 1:5 with water, producing a concentration of 10 mg/ml. An adult gerbil can be given 0.1 ml (1 mg) twice daily.

Tx 5. Trimethoprim/sulphonamide

Borgal 7.5% (Hoechst UK Ltd.)

This contains 12.5 mg/ml trimethoprim and 62.5 mg/ml sulphadoxine.

Dose: This can be given by subcutaneous injection at a dose of 0.1 ml daily.

Tx 6. Chlortetracycline

Aureomycin Ophthalmic Ointment (Cyanamid UK)

This contains 1% chlortetracycline hydrochloride.

Dose: Apply to the nose twice daily.

Probiotics

These can be given at the same time as antibiotics, or in times of debilitation, to improve the appetite.

Tx 7. Avipro (Vetark Health)

This is a water soluble probiotic, containing *Lactobacillus acidophilus*, *Enterococcus faecium* and *Saccharomyces* with electrolyes.

Dose: Avipro can be diluted in the drinking water at a rate of 5 g/200 ml water.

Comment: It is also useful in periods of stress, to protect the gastro-intestinal tract from stress-related disease.

Tx 8. Enterodex (Vydex Animal Health)

This contains the beneficial bacteria *Enterococcus*, similar to *Lactobacillus.*

Dose: One teaspoonful (5 g) in the drinking water is sufficient for 40 gerbils. For single gerbils a small pinch can be mixed with the drinking water.

Anti-fungal agents

Tx 9. Griseofulvin

Grisovin tablets (Mallinckrodt Veterinary Ltd.)

The tablets each contain 125 mg griseofulvin.

Dose: The dose is 25 mg/kg. Assuming that not all the dry food is ingested one quarter of a tablet can be safely crushed and sprinkled on the dry food daily, for 3–4 weeks. Griseofulvin should not be given during pregnancy because it may be teratogenic.

Tx 10. Povidone–iodine

Pevidine Antiseptic Solution (BK Veterinary Products)

Dose: This can be diluted 1:5 and used as a shampoo. Its effects are increased if the shampoo is left for 5 minutes before rinsing.

Tx 11. Chlorhexidine

Hibbiscrub (Pitman Moore)

This contains 4% w/v chlorhexidine; it is an antiseptic and bacteriostat. Although it has no antifungal properties, it may be a useful adjunct to therapy because of its antiseptic action.

Ectoparasitic preparations

Tx 12. Amitraz

Aludex (Hoechst UK Ltd.)

Aludex contains 50 g/litre amitraz.

Dose: The recommended concentration is 0.01% (100 ppm) amitraz; this is achieved by diluting 1 ml Aludex in 0.5 litre of water. The solution should be used as a dip, and not rinsed.

Tx 13. Ivermectin

Ivomec Injection for Cattle (Merck, Sharpe & Dohme Ltd.)

Ivomec contains 1% w/v ivermectin.

Dose: It can be given by subcutaneous injection at a dose rate of 200–400 µg/kg every 10 days. Ivomec can be diluted 1:10 with water and 0.02 ml given by injection.

Alternatively undiluted Ivomec can be given by mouth at a dose of 1 drop, repeated at 10 day intervals as necessary.

Ivermectin can be used in conjunction with Aludex (Tx 12) baths.

Endoparasitic preparations

Tx 14. Piperazine

Antepar Elixir (Wellcome)

Antepar contains 150 mg/ml piperazine, and will control nematodes (pinworms).

Dose: The required concentration of 2 mg/ml piperazine in the drinking water can be achieved by diluting the elixir 1:75 with water, and replacing the drinking water with this solution.

Tx 15. Niclosamide

Troscan 100 (Bayer plc)

These tablets each contain 100 mg niclosamide.

Dose: One tenth of a tablet can be given to an adult gerbil, and the dose repeated after 7 days.

Miscellaneous treatments

Tx 16. Corticosteroids

These are useful in cases of both endotoxic shock, and shock following trauma.

Dexadreson (Intervet UK Ltd.)

This contains a rapid action formulation of dexamethasone at a concentration of 2 mg/ml.

Dose: Dexadreson can be given by intramuscular injection at a dose of 0.03 ml.

Tx 17. Kaolin/pectin mixture

Kaogel (Parke Davis & Co Ltd.)

Kaogel contains 20% w/v light kaolin, and 0.43% w/v pectin. Many paediatric diarrhoea preparations are similar, and make suitable alternatives.

Dose: 0.1–0.2 ml orally three times daily, as an adjunct to other diarrhoea therapy.

Tx 18. Oral rehydration solution

Lectade (Pfizer Ltd.)

This contains dextrose monohydrate, sodium chloride, aminoacetic acid, potassium citrate and citric acid.

Dose: The liquid form can be diluted 20 ml lectade into 250 ml water, and given orally whenever fluid replacement is indicated.

Tx 19. Primidone

Mysoline (Mallinckrodt Veterinary Ltd.)

This contains 50 mg/ml primidone, and can be used to control seizures of any origin.

Dose: 0.05–0.1 ml given orally twice daily.

Tx 20. Megestrol acetate

Ovarid (Glaxo Ltd.)

May be used to reduce the activity of the sebaceous gland.

Dose: 1 mg on alternate days.

Eye preparations

Tx 21. Cepravin Eye Ointment (Mallinckrodt Veterinary Ltd.)

This contains a semisynthetic broad-spectrum bactericidal cephalosporin. It can be applied once daily.

Tx 22. Neobiotic HC (Upjohn Ltd.)

This contains the antibiotic neomycin and hydrocortisone as the steroid. It is a ready flowing liquid and can be applied two or three times daily.

Tx 23. Golden Eye Ointment (Typharm Ltd.)

This is available from pharmacists and contains dibromopropamidine isethionate 0.15% w/w and liquid paraffin. It is useful for minor eye infections and conjunctivitis. It can be applied once or twice daily.

HAMSTERS

Hamsters are one of the most popular small pets, having been kept as pets in Britain since 1945. There are over 20 species of hamster; the most commonly kept as a pet is the golden (Syrian) hamster *Mesocricetus auratus*. Also kept are the smaller Chinese hamster *Cricetulus griseus*, the Russian (Djungarian) hamster *Phodopus sungorus* (also known as the furry-footed hamster), and the Roborovski hamster *Phodopus roborovskii*. Nearly all the golden hamsters kept in captivity today are decendents of three hamsters which were brought over from Syria where they were found in a burrow by an archaeologist near Aleppo.

Hamsters are crepuscular animals (active at dawn and dusk) and Syrian hamsters are best kept singly. Russian hamsters can be kept in pairs, and Chinese hamsters can be kept in pairs or family groups. Russian hamsters prefer to be kept together, and a Russian kept alone may have a reduced lifespan; Chinese hamsters are not affected if kept singly.

10 HUSBANDRY AND NUTRITION

Housing

Hamsters are best kept in metal or plastic cages. The minimum cage size should be 60 cm × 30 cm × 23 cm (l × w × h). Cages should not be too tall, because the hamster can readily fracture limbs if it falls.

Cages can be made of wood, but must be strong enough to resist the hamster's persistent gnawing. Space can be increased by adding extra plywood shelves. Ventilation is important, and at least part of the cage should be made of wire. There are plastic cages available constructed of many tunnels and tubes, and whilst these are excellent for preventing boredom they must have adequate ventilation, or condensation can build up leading to damp bedding, they can also become very hot in warm weather.

Hamsters are escapologists and any cage needs to be secure. Dwarf hamsters are best kept in tanks, or cages with narrow bars usually sold for mice. Privacy is important, and exposed cages such as bird cages should not be used because they are too stressful.

The cage should be furnished with playthings, such as cardboard tubes, wooden nest boxes, and empty jam jars to prevent boredom and reduce stress.

An exercise wheel should be provided; the solid type is preferred because there is less risk of injury. However, with long haired hamsters care must be taken with any type of wheel, because they can easily catch their hair in the wheel axle. Wheels sold for mice are too small for hamsters and will lead to fur rubbing. Wire wheels can be converted to solid wheels with an insert of cardboard. If exercise is limited the hamster may appear stiff and reluctant to move. This condition is termed cage paralysis, and facilities for more exercise must be provided. Care must be taken when

109

using plastic exercise balls as the hamster cannot stop in them and may readily become exhausted.

Russian hamsters enjoy a dish of silver sand or budgie grit to roll in.

Bedding

Hamsters are avid nest builders and should be provided with plenty of bedding. Suitable bedding materials are sawdust, woodshavings, shredded paper and hay. Artificial fibre and cotton wool should be avoided because they may be ingested and cause impaction or constipation. The fibre can also become impacted in the cheek pouches and cause choking. Such fibre can also become wrapped around limbs or necks with fatal results.

Sawdust must not be too fine or dusty as it will trigger respiratory allergy and disease. Wood shavings are unsuitable for long-haired hamsters as they tend to tangle the coat. Long-haired hamsters should be kept on sawdust, or wood block cat litter.

White kitchen towel or plain white paper are suitable bedding materials, but newspaper and coloured paper are not, because printing inks are extremely toxic to hamsters.

If hay is given it must be dry, and free from dust and parasites.

Environment

The cage must be kept out of direct sunlight, and not too close to a heat source, e.g. radiator. It must be sited away from draughts. Hamsters can withstand cold better than heat providing they have plenty of bedding. Dwarf hamsters are particularly susceptible to heat stroke. The room temperature should be between 18 and 21°C (64–70°F) with a relative humidity of 40–60%.

Breeders with large numbers of hamsters prefer to keep them in a separate unit, a room, shed or garage. If using a garage, the car should be kept outside as exhaust fumes are poisonous. The unit should be kept at a constant temperature; it should be insulated and heated during the winter months. There must be plenty of ventilation in the summer; if using a shed, air vents can be fitted at either end. The unit should not be in direct sunlight, because during the summer the temperature can increase rapidly leading to fatal heat stroke. The roof can be painted white to reflect the heat and keep the building cool.

Predators such as dogs and cats, and wild birds and rodents must be excluded, particularly as they may carry disease. Insects should also be excluded, and the more old-fashioned dichlorvos-impregnated (Vapona) sticky strips are the safest method of doing this. These strips are also thought to reduce ectoparasite numbers.

Stocking

Syrian hamsters

Adult golden hamsters must be housed separately. Youngsters can live together until they are 6–8 weeks of age and then fighting will break out. The only exception is males that have been kept together since weaning, but even these may become aggressive. Females will not live together, and may not even live with a male for long. Females will generally only accept a male when they are in oestrus, and then only for a short period.

Russian hamsters

Dwarf Russian hamsters are more social animals than Syrian hamsters, living in family groups in the wild; they may live more readily in pairs in captivity. Pairs should be introduced to each other when young, although an older male may accept a younger female (not vice versa). Two Russian hamsters of the same sex will usually live together without fighting.

Chinese hamsters

Chinese hamsters are less sociable than Russian hamsters, but can be kept in pairs or small groups if introduced when young.

Roborovski hamsters

Roborovski hamsters are best kept as pairs and not in colonies.

Hygiene

Cages must be cleaned weekly. As the hamster is a habitual hoarder, the store of food must be checked daily, and anything that is damp or mouldy removed. After cleaning, part of the previous nest can be replaced in the cage. Hamsters may often reserve one corner of the cage for toileting and this should be cleaned daily. It is also possible to place a shallow container or jam jar in this corner which they will use as a litter tray.

Nutrition and feeding

Hamsters are excellent hoarders, and they possess elasticated cheek pouches in which they can carry large quantities of food and bedding. The name hamster comes from the German word hamstern which means to hoard! They are best fed once daily in the early evening, before their peak of activity. The food should be provided in a hopper or heavy dish to prevent spillage and faecal contamination.

Dry food

Proprietary hamster mixes contain mixed corn, maize, alfalfa, dried peas, sunflower seeds and peanuts. Mixed bird seed, suitable for canaries and small cage birds, can also be added to the dry food, especially for dwarf hamsters. An average dry food intake is 5–7 g daily. An excess of sunflower seeds may lead to obesity and calcium deficiency, because they are high in fat and low in calcium. Peanuts are very high in protein and an excess may lead to coat changes and digestive disturbances. The dry food should not contain any sharp husks which could damage the pouch linings.

Weaning

Hamsters will start eating solid food at 7–10 days old. Weaning is complete at 21–25 days of age. After the age of 3 weeks very small quantities of vegetables such as carrots, celery, spinach and parsley should be given to supplement the diet. Fruit such as apples, pears and bananas can also be introduced. Youngsters that are fed a varied diet from an early age are less likely to get digestive upsets later in life. No green food should be introduced in excess or fed in exclusion because dietary diarrhoea will develop. Frosted food or food direct from the refrigerator should not be given because it will cause digestive upset.

Green food

In adults the feeding of green food is useful in preventing obesity. Green food must be fed dry because wet green food will result in an increased water intake, and subsequent loose faeces. Small quantities of fruit and vegetables can be given daily (see Weaning). Fresh wild plants such as yarrow, chickweed, groundsel, dandelion and young raspberry leaves can also be offered in small quantities. Dandelion is a laxative, whereas raspberry leaves, yarrow and shepherd's purse have astringent qualities.

Protein

In their natural state hamsters eat earthworms and mealworms. They can be offered small quantities of cat and dog food, or raw beef and mutton (not pork) although these may be too high in protein for the older animal. There is no evidence that feeding meat increases the incidence of cannibalism.

Protein in the form of hard-boiled eggs and cheese can be given occasionally, and is useful for pregnant and nursing females. Powdered baby milk can be sprinkled on the dry food, in the nest, and on young of 4–5 days old; the mother and the young will lick at the powder and obtain useful protein. Nursing females and their young can also be given milk in the form of baby cereals, or milk-soaked bread.

The protein content for young and breeding females should be 24%.

Forbidden foods

Hamsters will attempt to eat and hoard anything. They must not be given junk food snacks such as cake or sweets. Sticky sweets will cause pouch impaction, and chocolate ingestion will lead to death, due to the toxic effects of the alkaloid theobromine which it contains.

Gnawing

Hamsters need a supply of food to gnaw to prevent incisor overgrowth. The nuts in the dry mix will help; dog biscuits and wholewheat macaroni can be provided. Bread can also be baked and used for gnawing. Wood from non-poisonous trees can be provided and apple branches are a particular favourite.

Water

Fresh water should be available at all times, preferably from a drinking bottle, because dishes are easily soiled.

On average an adult will consume 15–20 ml water a day. The nozzle of the bottle is best made of stainless steel as it will resist gnawing: hamsters can damage aluminium. The water bottles must be cleaned regularly, because if green algae are allowed to build up they can cause diarrhoea. Leaking sipper bottles can cause alopecia if the hamster regularly becomes wettened.

It is important that the sipper bottle is accessible to all the hamsters, and low enough for any babies to reach.

Vitamins

The process of eating its own droppings (coprophagy) is normal in the adult hamster, and the redigestion of these faeces satisfies the requirement for vitamins B and K. These vitamins are formed by the bacterial flora, and redigested as copraphagy occurs.

11 SYSTEMS AND DISEASES

THE SKIN

Scent glands

Hamsters possess two scent glands, known as hip spots, one on either flank. They appear as a dark discolouration of the skin, which may be greasy. They are most prominent in the male, but are quite normal. They are most noticeable in the breeding season, and the male may lick the glands so that they appear wet and bald; however, no treatment is required unless they become severely inflamed, and then castration could be considered. Dwarf hamsters also possess a ventral scent gland.

Neoplasms of the scent glands do occur in the older hamster, the commonest being melanomas and haemangiosarcomas.

If male hamsters are kept together they may cannibalise each other's glands.

Sores inside legs

This is a common problem and occurs when the hamster uses a wire (non-solid) exercise wheel. The hamster puts its legs through the bars and spokes, and rubs the fur from its legs. The wheel should be changed or converted to the solid type with an insert of strong cardboard. The sores can be bathed and treated with a suitable cream, e.g. Dermisol (Tx 21).

Ringworm

This is generally caused by *Trichophyton mentagrophytes*, but also by *Trichophyton simii*, *Microsporum canis* and *Microsporum gypseum*.

115

Fungal infections may be more common in the enclosed plastic type of cages, as in these the development of condensation allows the bedding to become damp, a suitable environment for fungi to survive.

Clinical signs: These include alopecia, and dry skin with yellow, flaky seborrhoea. The body and ear pinnae are affected. The condition is sometimes pruritic.

Diagnosis: Microscopy, and culture on Saburaud's medium should be carried out.

Treatment: The patient should be handled with gloves and may be washed with a povidone–iodine shampoo (Tx 11) or an anti-fungal preparation such as natamycin (Tx 10. Mycophyt). If possible the hair should be clipped before shampooing. Griseofulvin (Tx 9) may be given at a dose rate of 25 mg/kg for at least 3 weeks. The cage should be cleaned out with povidone-iodine solution (Tx 11).

The ventilation in the cage should be improved, and if the nest box is made of plastic the lid can be removed.

Demodecosis

The causal agents are *Demodex criceti* and *Demodex aurati*. Infection with these mites is common, but clinical disease is only seen if the immune system is compromised, in the young, pregnant or aged.

Clinical signs: These include dry alopecia, some papules and scaling.

Diagnosis: Microscopy of skin scrapings is necessary.

Treatment: Ivermectin 1% w/v (Tx 13. Ivomec Injection for Cattle) can be given undiluted orally. One drop is given, and repeated every 10 days as necessary. Weekly amitraz baths (Tx 12) are also effective.

Sarcoptic mange

Clinical signs: There is hairloss around the face which is pruritic. The condition is contagious.

Diagnosis: Microscopy to reveal the mite *Sarcoptes scabiei* is necessary.

Treatment: Ivermectin 1% w/v (Tx 13) can be given orally every 10 days for a month.

Fleas

Ctenocephalides can be transmitted from dogs and cats in the same household. The hamster can be dusted with a pyrethrin powder or spray (Tx 14. Johnsons Anti-mite Spray for Birds), or treated with fipronil (Tx 15. Frontline) at a dose of 7.5 mg/kg.

Alopecia

Generalised hair loss can also be seen in the geriatric hamster related to chronic renal failure, or an endocrine neoplasm. Both Cushing's disease and hypothyroidism are recognised and may cause hair loss and coat thinning. Hair loss may also be associated with rubbing on the exercise wheel, a feeder or leaking drinker, or any abrasive bedding. Alopecia has also been recorded in hamsters bedded on shavings made from treated wood. Hair loss can be associated with low protein diets containing less than 16% protein.

Non-specific alopecia is often improved by adding one or two drops of cod-liver oil to the diet, daily. Proprietary products, e.g. Vitapet Small Animal Fur Conditioner, containing cod-liver oil and vitamins A and D, can also be used. The addition of a yeast tablet crushed on the food daily may also be beneficial.

Hair loss may also be associated with a diet high in overheating cereals. This can be improved by feeding more fruit and vegetables, and by substituting half the dry ration with boiled rice or puffed rice cereal.

Thin hair-coat associated with satinisation

The Satin gene (Sa) produces a shiny deep coloured coat. Satins should always be mated to normal coated hamsters. In a Satin × Satin mating the offspring have a thin hair coat (supersatinisation). If Supersatins interbreed the resultant offspring are bald with only a thin covering of fine hairs.

Pyoderma and abscesses

Pyoderma is generally caused by *Staphylococcus aureus* as a result of fighting, or through abrasions in the skin. Infected bite wounds will develop into abscesses. Other pathogens include *Streptococcus* spp. and *Pasteurella pneumotropica*.

Treatment: Antibiotics (Tx 1–6) can be given orally and used topically. The wounds should be cleaned with an antibacterial wash. Dermisol liquid (Tx 21) is a useful cleansing agent. Abscesses may need to be regularly lanced and drained.

Allergic dermatitis

Clinical signs: Skin lesions form part of a range of allergy symptoms, which may also include sneezing and an ocular discharge, and swollen feet. The skin is seborrhoeic, with white flakes particularly around the eyes and ears. There may be some generalised hair loss.

Causes: The allergens are usually food or bedding. However, some hamsters may be allergic to cigarette smoke, hair or furniture polish, or perfume, and these factors should be considered.

Treatment: The bedding should be changed, If sawdust or woodshavings have been used, these should be replaced with shredded white paper. Synthetic bedding can be replaced with meadow hay.

Foods that should be eliminated from the diet are sunflower seeds and peanuts. Any coloured biscuit pieces (containing dyes with E numbers) should also be removed. The diet can be altered to include cooked rice, fruit and maizeflakes.

THE REPRODUCTIVE SYSTEM

Litter size: 6–8
Birth weight: 2–5 g
Weaning age: 21–25 days
Fur grows: 5 days
Eyes open: 10-12 days
Puberty: 45–60 days
Best age to breed: Males 10–14 weeks
                          female 12–14 weeks
Breeding life: 1 year (5–7 litters possible, ideally 2–3)
Oestrus: every 4 days
Post-partum oestrus: infertile
Gestation: Golden 16–18 days
                 Russian 18–20 days
                 Chinese 21 days

Sexing

The anogenital distance is larger in the male than the female. In the male it is also possible to see the scrotal sacs, and the testicles can be made to protrude by gentle pressure on the abdomen (Figure 11.1). Hamsters possess scent glands on their flanks; these are most prominent in the male and are seen as patches of darkened skin which may be greasy.

The female has seven pairs of nipples on her abdomen, which are visible even in the young female. The majority of male hamsters have no nipples.

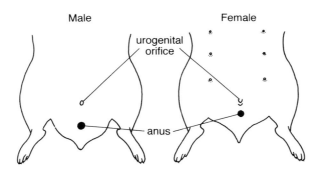

Figure 11.1 External genitalia.

Breeding

Although females are capable of breeding from 6 or 8 weeks of age it is best to leave them until 12 weeks unless they are very mature. Some breeders prefer to wait until the female is 4–6 months old before her first mating. Females come into oestrus every fourth day, usually in the late evening, generally 30–60 minutes after nightfall.

Pairing and mating

Syrian hamsters: When pairing Syrian hamsters the female must always be put in with the male and not vice versa. If a male is put in with the female she may attack him even if she is in oestrus. Alternatively they can both be placed in a neutral mating cage or box. The hamsters should be paired in the late evening. A female Syrian hamster will only accept a male whilst she is in oestrus, and then only for a short period of time. If she is aggressive towards him they must be separated immediately, and the pairing repeated on subsequent nights. If she is in oestrus and receptive she will adopt the classic posture for mating, crouched down with her body and legs extended and her tail in the air (lordosis). She may adopt a similar posture if gently stroked along her back. The male will then repeatedly mount her and mating may last for 10 minutes. The pair should then be separated, as the female will become aggressive.

Chinese hamsters: Chinese hamsters can be kept as breeding pairs or family groups. When they are kept together the first sign that the female is pregnant is often her aggression towards the male. Although she may initially exclude the male after parturition, he may be allowed to help as the youngsters grow. In a group situation of Chinese hamsters only the dominant female may breed, or she may take the young from other females and rear them herself.

Russian hamsters: These can be kept as breeding pairs or family groups. If Russian hamsters are paired, both male and female are involved in the upbringing of the youngsters, and the young tend to develop best when brought up by both parents.

Pregnancy diagnosis

Before ovulation the female will have a thin clear discharge from her vulva. After mating this discharge becomes opaque, thick and sticky (the copulatory plug).

Some breeders like to perform a 'check mating' 4 days after the original mating. If the female refuses the male she is probably pregnant. However it is not infallible, and some pregnant females may accept the male, whilst some non-pregnant females may reject him.

A pregnant female will develop a noticeable abdominal swelling by 9–10 days' gestation.

Pseudopregnancy

Pseudopregnancy can last 7–13 days and follows an infertile mating. Usually the female will look swollen 10 days after mating and if she does not she is either carrying a small litter or is pseudopregnant. If it is the latter she can be paired with the male on day 12–14 as she is likely to return to oestrus.

Gestation

Gestation lasts 16–18 days in the golden hamster, 18-20 days in the Russian, and 21 days in the Chinese hamster. From day 13 the female should not be handled, and she should be disturbed as little as possible. A large supply of nesting material (hay and shredded white paper) and food should be offered at this time, and she should be left alone. Hamsters are avid nest builders, and this process may stimulate the hormones for parturition and lactation.

During gestation the female should be given extra protein such as egg, cheese and milk.

Delayed implantation is possible, resulting in apparently longer gestation times.

Parturition

It is sensible to have the hamster in a solid-sided cage during parturition and rearing of the young, because the babies could be accidently pushed through the bars of a mesh cage.

Before parturition the female will become restless and have a bloody discharge from the vulva; birth soon follows. Parturition generally takes place at night. The young are born naked, pink and with their eyes closed. Unlike other rodents they are born with their incisor teeth. If the female is disturbed at this stage she can pick up her litter in her cheek pouches without harming them.

A female may abandon or cannibalise her young if she is disturbed, if the nest is scant or if there is too little food and water. If the litter is very large or if the female develops agalactia she may cannibalise some of the young. The female should not be disturbed for 10 days other than to provide fresh food and bedding.

Females have a post-partum oestrus which lasts for 5 hours after the birth, and which is infertile. Their next fertile oestrus is usually 2–18 days post-weaning. However, a female should be allowed to recover from her first litter for 2–3 months before remating to enable her to regain her condition. Although the female has a breeding potential of 7–9 litters in her breeding life it is fairer to restrict her to two or three litters.

If parturition has not occurred after 18 days (Syrian hamster), 20 days (Russian) or 21 days (Chinese) it may be necessary to consider inducing the birth with 0.5 i.u. oxytocin.

Weaning

The young become furred at 5 days of age and their eyes open at around 10 days, when they also start eating solid food, nibbling at pieces that the female brings back to the nest. Bread and milk can be provided at this time, but the young are able to manage small pieces of hamster mix.

The young should be separated from the female by 3–4 weeks, because she may start to attack them after this time. The young must be sexed and separated from each other by 6 weeks otherwise they will start to inter-breed.

Problems after parturition

Fostering

Fostering is unsuccessful, and the foster mother may cannibalise her own young as well as the foster litter. The young are too immature to hand rear.

Mastitis

Clinical signs: Mastitis usually occurs when the young are 7–10 days old. The affected glands are warm and swollen with a haemorrhagic discharge. Often the female will cannibalise her young. This is commonly associated with β-haemolytic streptococcal infection.

Treatment: Antibiotic therapy (Tx 1–6) should be carried out, preferably based on culture and sensitivity tests.

Infertility

The female

- A female will fail to breed if she is overweight. Her weight can be reduced by introducing more green food, and less concentrated mix. A female which is not bred from whilst young has more time to become obese and hence infertile.
- Hamsters are seasonal breeders; as day length decreases litters become smaller, neonatal mortality increases, and breeding stops altogether. In the winter the female becomes anoestrus and the male's testes may retract. The breeding season can be artificially extended by providing

14–18 daylight hours with electric light, and maintaining an environmental temperature of 22–24°C (72–75°F).

- Rarely, females may be permanently anoestrus.
- Young females may be inexperienced; they should be paired with an experienced male.
- Roborovski hamsters are harder to breed than the other species, and they have higher dietary protein requirements. Their diet should be supplemented with eggs, meat and mealworms. Other hamsters may also be fed an increased protein ration during the breeding season to enhance fertility.
- Albino Chinese hamsters tend to be infertile.
- Russian and Chinese hamsters that live in colonies may be infertile because of their social ranking; a dominant female may breed regularly, whilst more submissive females may have suppressed fertility.

The male

- Stud males may become infertile if they are overused. Ideally, males should only be used once or twice weekly, and given a short rest every month. Stud males also benefit from vitamin E supplementation, which can be achieved by sprinkling wheatgerm on their dry food. Both sexes should be fed an increased protein ration in the breeding season.
- If the environmental temperature is low the male's testicles may retract, or he may penetrate the female but not have enough fertile sperm. He should be kept at an increased temperature for at least a week before mating again.
- Overweight males will become infertile.

Ovarian cysts

These are common in females that are not bred from. The clinical signs are a swollen abdomen and a bloody vaginal discharge. The cysts can contain as much as 2 ml of follicular fluid. The cysts are usually bilateral. They can be drained by paracentesis, or ovariohysterectomy can be performed.

Pyometra

Pyometras have also been recorded; treatment with antibiotics may provide temporary relief, or ovariohysterectomy can be attempted.

Pyometra can be a sequel to respiratory infection with *Streptococcus* spp. and *Pasteurella pneumotropica*. Lymphocytic choriomeningitis virus (LCMV) can also cause pyometra and infertility.

Testicular tumours

These are recognised in the older male as firm enlargements of the testicles, which may lead to discomfort. Castration is curative.

THE URINARY SYSTEM

Physiology

Normal hamster urine is opaque, thick and yellow, of pH 8. It contains small crystals and it should not be mistaken for pus. On the day following oestrus females produce a similar vaginal discharge which is normal.

URINARY TRACT DISORDERS

Urolithiasis

Clinical signs: These include polydipsia, polyuria, dysuria and haematuria. The uroliths may be palpable.

Treatment: Cystotomy to remove the urolith may be necessary. Due to the nature of the urine there is a tendency for the stones to recur.

Renal amyloidosis and chronic renal failure

Clinical signs: Polydipsia, polyuria and haematuria are seen. Geriatric hamsters also develop hair loss and sticky eyes. Amyloidosis may affect the adrenal glands. Renal failure is a common sequel to sleeper disease (heat stroke), due to the dehydration caused.

Treatment: Reduction of dietary protein may help. Cooked rice can be given, and the protein level of the dried food reduced by mixing in 50% puffed rice cereal. If concurrent infection is suspected antibiotics can be given. In cases of renal failure following heat stroke fluid replacement is very important and oral rehydration solution (Tx 24. Lectade) is recommended for this purpose.

THE DIGESTIVE SYSTEM

Physiology

Coprophagy is part of the normal digestive process, enabling the hamster to ingest valuable B vitamins formed by the microflora of the caecum. The stomach of the hamster has two compartments, a non-glandular fore-stomach (equivalent to the rumen) where some pre-gastric fermentation takes place, and a glandular stomach.

The hamster also possesses two elastic cheek pouches which are thin walled and highly distensible. The lining of these pouches is made up of stratified epithelium and is quite dry, resulting in impaction if sticky foods are hoarded.

DIGESTIVE SYSTEM DISORDERS

The teeth

Malocclusion

Malocclusion of the incisor teeth may occur if a tooth is broken by a fall or on a feeder, and the remaining teeth wear unevenly. Hamsters that gnaw their cage bars are also likely to break teeth. Affected hamsters will have difficulty eating, and may become polydipsic.

The teeth can be clipped level, and hard food such as dog biscuits, wholewheat macaroni and nuts can be given to encourage gnawing. For tooth clipping it is easiest to restrain the hamster in a towel encompassing the body and feet.

The teeth may break more easily if the diet is low in calcium. An excess of sunflower seeds will lead to calcium deficiency. Dog biscuits are a good source of calcium and phosphorus and hamsters with weak teeth can be given supplementary calcium in the form of milk or cheese. If the mal-occlusion is such that gnawing is difficult, the hamster can be given softer foods such as porridge, mashes or baby cereal.

Malocclusion can also be congenital. Hamsters are born with fully erupted incisor teeth, and if these grow unevenly clipping may be required as frequently as once a week.

Dental caries

Dental caries are common; their presence is related to the amount of treats and table snacks that are fed. High carbohydrate and high acid diets cause an increased incidence of dental caries. Caries can progress to tooth root abscesses, with associated salivation, facial swelling and anorexia. Tooth extraction is possible, together with antibiosis (Tx 1–6).

The mouth

Foreign bodies lodged between the teeth may cause dysphagia and abscesses in the mouth. Increased salivation may be the first obvious symptom and the mouth should be examined carefully.

The cheek pouches

The pouch lining is dry epithelium, and care must be taken not to feed abrasive foods such as sharp seeds and oat husks because they will readily damage the pouches.

Impaction

The cheek pouches can become impacted with sticky foods such as sweets. Abscesses can also develop due to infection with *Streptococcus* spp. and *Staphylococcus aureus*. Both impaction and infection will present with clinical signs of salivation, anorexia and facial swelling.

Diagnosis: Needle aspiration of the swelling will differentiate between impaction and abscessation.

Treatment: The glands should be flushed out with water or an antibacterial preparation. Antibiotics (Tx 1–6) should be administered for abscessation.

Eversion

The cheek pouches can become everted in dwarf Russian and Chinese hamsters. Eversion can be readily replaced. If the pouch is everted long enough for it to become necrotic, surgical resection is necessary.

The stomach and intestines

Diarrhoea associated with dietary change

Clinical signs: Loose droppings, soiling of the vent area and cage. In the early stages the hamster remains bright and will still eat.

Treatment: This consists of removal of all food, except the dry mix. The hamster can be offered burnt toast, or fed a small amount of charcoal crushed with water throu.,n a syringe or eye-dropper. Boiled rice, and arrowroot biscuits or powdered arrowroot can be given. Kaolin/pectin mixtures (Tx 19) can also be administered. Green food should only be reintroduced 3–4 days after the diarrhoea has resolved.

Comment: If the water bottles are not cleaned regularly, and green algae are allowed to build up, this can also cause diarrhoea.

'Wet tail' (proliferative ileitis)

This is also known as transmissible ileal hyperplasia. It is a multifactorial disease associated with stresses such as weaning (3–5 weeks of age) and changes of environment, such as the move from pet shop to new home. Malnutrition and overcrowding are also predisposing factors. Colibacillosis has been implicated as a cause of this disease, but in some cases it may be a secondary pathogen. *Campylobacter* spp. have also been identified as a factor in this disease. Hamsters may also carry *Cryptosporidia* spp. in their intestines.

The pathogens are spread by the faecal–oral route between weanlings, or from adult to weanling.

The disease is seen most frequently in long-haired varieties; there may be some familial predisposition. Wet tail is rare in dwarf hamsters.

Clinical signs: The acute form causes severe watery diarrhoea and soiling of the vent. The hamster adopts a hunched position and is lethargic and anorexic, and death from dehydration occurs within 2–3 days. The more chronic form will lead to intussception, or rectal prolapse. Peritonitis may also develop.

Pathology: At necropsy the intestines, especially the ileum, are congested and oedematous. The gut contents are yellow, mucoid and often bloody. The mesenteric lymph nodes are enlarged.

Treatment: This may be unsuccessful in severe cases; supportive therapy and nursing are aimed at reducing stress and correcting dehydration.

The hamster should be kept in warm, clean surroundings; an airing cupboard provides an ideal environment.

Dehydration can be corrected by administering warmed fluids, either lactated Ringer's solution (Tx 22), or 5% glucose–saline (Tx 23). The maximum amount for fluid replacement is 3 ml (subcutaneous injection) and 3 ml (intraperitoneal injection). Oral rehydration solution (Tx 24. Lectade) can be given. Fluids only should be given for the first 24 hours; solid food should be witheld.

Kaolin/pectin mixtures (Tx 19. Kaogel) can be administered by mouth at a dose of two or three drops three times a day.

Antibiotics such as neomycin (Tx 4) or metronidazole (Tx 3) can be given.

Other supportive measures include injections of multivitamins, especially vitamin B, and an injection of corticosteroids (Tx 18), to combat shock. Vitamin B can also be given in the form of brewer's yeast.

Prevention: Good husbandry and hygiene are necessary, with frequent bedding changes. Removal of all stress factors is required. Both oxytetracycline (Tx 5) and erythromycin (Tx 2) have been added to the drinking water to control outbreaks in colonies.

Oxytetracycline (Tx 5) can be added to the drinking water at a dose rate of 400 mg/litre, and erythromycin (Tx 2) can be used with care at 100 mg/litre.

If the hamster dies the bedding must be destroyed and the cage thoroughly disinfected before repopulating with another hamster. All food dishes and water bottles must also be disinfected.

Antibiotic induced diarrhoea

The administration of some antibiotics alters the intestinal microflora in a way which allows proliferation of *Clostridium* spp., particularly *Clostridium difficile*. This proliferation produces enterotoxins which cause fatal enteritis and diarrhoea. The most toxic drugs are those which have a narrow spectrum of activity against Gram-positive organisms, e.g. erythromycin, penicillin, lincomycin, cephalosporin and streptomycin.

Broad spectrum antibiotics are safer, and enrofloxacin, tetracycline, metronidazole and neomycin are recommended. When using an antibiotic, concurrent administration of a probiotic (Tx 7 and 8), and additional vitamin B is suggested.

Salmonellosis

Salmonella spp. may cause subclinical disease, manifesting as a loss of condition, or they may cause diarrhoea. The causal agents are *Salmonella enteriditis* and *Salmonella typhimurium*. This disease is a zoonosis.

Tyzzer's disease

This is caused by the organism *Bacillus piliformis* and is seen in weanling hamsters, or stressed individuals, particularly if they are associated with mice. Infective spores can survive for up to a year in bedding, soil or contaminated feed.

Clinical signs: There is acute diarrhoea, and death within 24 hours associated with dehydration. A more chronic wasting disease may also be seen.

Diagnosis: At necropsy yellow/grey foci are seen on the liver which are 1–2 mm in diameter; the intestines are oedematous and haemorrhagic. There may also be white foci on the myocardium.
   Bacillus piliformis may be detectable on liver smears.

Treatment: This is generally unsuccessful in acute cases, but supportive therapy, fluids, warmth and nursing can be tried (see 'Wet tail').
   Medication with oxytetracycline (Tx 5) can be attempted to reduce the extent of an outbreak using a dilution of 400 mg/litre in the drinking water for 10 days. A lower dilution of 100 mg/litre for 30 days has also been reported.

Yersinia

Clinical signs: The acute form is a septicaemia, and sudden death. The chronic form, which is more common, is seen as weight loss, anorexia and chronic diarrhoea. It is caused by *Yersinia pseudotuberculosis* which is spread by the faeces of wild birds and rodents.

Diagnosis: At necropsy there are abscesses and necrosis in the mesenteric lymph nodes, the liver and spleen, and the organism can be cultured from these areas.

Treatment: This is not recommended because yersinia is a zoonosis. Affected animals should be culled, and the premises thoroughly disinfected. Wild birds and rodents should be kept away from the hamstery.

Intussusception

Hamsters are prone to this condition following any type of gut hypermotility, e.g. diarrhoea, 'wet tail', or the eating of laxative plants. Intussusception can follow impaction with dry food or unsuitable bedding material.

Clinical signs: There is a bloody diarrhoea, with severe abdominal discomfort which may progress to prolapse of the colon and rectum.

Treatment: Surgery could be attempted but is unlikely to be successful.

Rectal prolapse

This follows a period of diarrhoea, and is a sequel to intussusception. Replacement is generally unsuccessful, but can be attempted using a well lubricated thermometer if the exposed colon is clean. Corticosteroids (Tx 18) and fluids should be administered to combat shock. Rectal prolapse and 'wet tail' are infrequently seen in the Russian hamster.

Impaction (constipation)

This occurs if the hamster is fed dry food with no access to water, or if it ingests cotton wool or other artificial fibres. Weanling hamsters are prone to the condition, often as they start eating solids, and may not have full access to the sipper bottle. Lack of exercise may predispose to this condition. Endoparasitism can also cause constipation.

Clinical signs: There is abdominal discomfort, a swollen, discoloured abdomen and protruding anus. The hamster adopts a posture with an arched back. The hamster may pass only scant, small hard droppings.

Treatment: Very small doses of laxative can be given, taking care to avoid inducing hypermotility which would cause a progression to intussusception or rectal prolapse. One or two drops of syrup of figs, liquid paraffin or undiluted olive oil can be given three times daily from an eye dropper, or a laxative such as lactulose (Tx 25).

Laxative plants which can be given include dandelion leaves, groundsel and lettuce. The last provides the necessary extra fluid which is lacking in these cases. Small quantities of these plants should be included in the diet for a few days once the constipation has cleared.

Another remedy is to add a pinch of Epsom salts to the drinking water.

Endoparasites

Hymenolepis nana

Hymenolepis nana is also referred to as the dwarf tapeworm, and although infestation in hamsters is common it is usually without clinical signs. Infrequently it may cause a catarrhal enteritis and weight loss. It may also be responsible for impaction and constipation. It is a zoonosis.

Diagnosis: The hooked ova are present in the faeces. The adult tapeworm are found in the small intestine, and occasionally in the bile and pancreatic ducts.

Treatment: 100 mg/kg niclosamide (Tx 17) can be given orally and the dose repeated after 7 days. Troscan 100 tablets each contain 100 mg niclosamide and one tenth of a tablet can be crushed and administered to an adult hamster.

Transmission: Hymenolepis nana has both direct and indirect life cycles. In the direct life cycle ova are passed in the faeces from one host to another rodent host. Tissue migration occurs in the second host. Auto-infection is also possible, when the ova mature in the first host and undergo tissue migration.

In the indirect life cycle tissue migration does not occur. The ova are passed from the faeces of one rodent host, though an invertebrate (beetles or fleas) to another rodent host.

Prevention: Wild rodents and insects must be excluded from the surrounding environment. Food should be protected from contamination, and all bedding should be changed weekly. The ova survive longer in the environment if the humidity is high, and if this is the case the humidity should be lowered. Any in-contact dogs and cats should be wormed regularly.

Syphacia obvelata

Infection with this pinworm is common, but asymptomatic.

Diagnosis: The ova which are present in the faeces are banana shaped. They can be collected from the perineum using sticky tape.

Treatment: Piperazine citrate (Tx 16) can be given at a dose of 20 mg daily for an adult hamster for 7 days. Antepar Elixir contains 150 mg/ml and can be given undiluted at a dose of 0.13 ml daily, or it can be diluted 1:75 with the drinking water and administered in the water bottle.

Protozoa

Many protozoa have been recorded in hamsters, although none are thought to be pathogenic. These include *Balantidium* spp., *Cryptosporidium* and *Giardia*.

THE RESPIRATORY SYSTEM

Respiratory infections

Hamsters are susceptible to draughts and sudden falls in external temperature. They are able to contract common colds and influenza viruses from humans, particularly school children, and infection may lead to fatal pneumonia. *Pasteurella pneumotropica* is commonly carried by healthy hamsters, but may cause secondary infection if the hamster is stressed. *Streptococcus* spp. are frequently transmitted from humans.

Clinical signs: There is sneezing, with an ocular and nasal discharge. The hamster is lethargic, sits hunched with a rough coat and half closed eyes. It will often sit in a corner and shiver. The nose may become sore due to constant rubbing. The affected animal is pyrexic (up to 38°C (101°F)). Unless the hamster develops a secondary bacterial infection it will recover in 5–7 days.

Cases that recover may develop otitis media, with head tilt and ataxia after 7 days. Both *Pasteurella* and *Streptococcus* infections may also cause abscess formation in other sites, particularly the uterus, leading to abortions and infertility.

Treatment: Supportive nursing, and the provision of warmth, fluids and antibiotics are required. Enrofloxacin (Tx 1. Baytril) or a trimethoprim/sulphonamide preparation (Tx 6. Borgal 7.5%) are recommended.

The hamster can be given warm milk and water (1:1) with a little honey to drink. Mentholated ointment (e.g. Vick or Olbas oil) can be applied around the cage, or a very small amount dabbed on the hamster's chest.

Human decongestant containing 6 mg/ml pseudoephedrine hydrochloride (Tx 20. Sudafed), can be given at a dose of 1 drop twice daily.

Allergic rhinitis

Hamsters can become allergic to food, or more commonly bedding. Fine sawdust can produce both ocular and nasal irritation. Other causes are cigarette smoke, furniture polish and hair sprays. Allergies may be hereditary.

Clinical signs: Sneezing and ocular discharge occur, but otherwise the animal is healthy. Affected individuals are active and eat normally. Hair loss and sore feet may be accompanying symptoms.

Treatment: The bedding should be changed, all sawdust and synthetic material should be removed, and replaced with shredded white paper. Aerosols should not be used in the hamster's environment. Where food allergy is suspected the hamster should be fed an exclusion diet of boiled rice, white bread, vegetables, fruit and maizeflakes.

Dyspnoea associated with cardiac disease

Cardiac thrombosis secondary to degenerative cardiomyopathy or cardiac amyloidosis, may present as dyspnoea in older hamsters. The hamster will become tired very easily, and may collapse after using the exercise wheel; the extremities may become cyanotic.

The hamster is best housed in a cage where it cannot climb, e.g. in a glass or plastic aquarium, and the exercise wheel should be removed. Sunflower seeds, which have a high fat content should be removed from the diet.

THE EYE

Ocular discharge

This may be a symptom of respiratory infection, or allergic conjunctivitis. It may also be caused by a foreign body (usually fine sawdust) in the eye. Hamsters can also suffer from entropion.

Draughts will also cause an ocular discharge, as can exposure to a build up of ammonia from urine.

Clinical signs: These include a discharge from one or both eyes, conjunctivitis, or sticky eyes which do not open after sleep.

Treatment: If ocular discharge is a symptom of allergy or respiratory infection, these conditions should be treated. A foreign body can be flushed out with water. Antibiotic eye ointment containing chloramphenicol (Tx 26. Chloromycetin) can be applied twice daily for 5 days. If there is no corneal damage antibiotic/corticosteroid preparations can be used (Tx 27 and 28). Golden Eye Ointment (Tx 29) is another alternative for minor eye conditions.

Cases of entropion may require longer term antibiotic therapy, and as the condition is hereditary, affected animals should be removed from the breeding stock.

Glaucoma

This is seen most frequently in Campbells, and presents as a swelling of the globe and an increase in intraocular pressure. If the condition is uncomfortable, or the eye prolapses enucleation can be considered.

Glaucoma is thought to be an inherited condition, and affected hamsters should not be used for breeding.

Eye prolapse

Prolapse of the eye or rupture of the globe follow injuries from fighting. The eye becomes dry, and will usually heal sufficiently to make surgical intervention and enucleation unnecessary. Antibiotics (Tx 1–6) should be given for the first 5–7 days.

Microphthalmia

Congenitally small eyes, or anophthalmia may be present in some pure white hamsters, and are the result of a recessive gene. These hamsters should not be bred from, but are able to survive once they are familiar with their environment.

The white anophthalmic gene (Wh) is semi-lethal and carried by some strains of black-eyed white hamsters (black-eyed cream roans), some

Dominant spots and all white-bellied hamsters (Whwh). The breeding of the latter is discouraged because 25% of all offspring will have anophthalmia (WhWh). Roans also carry the gene (Whwh) and should not be mated together. Also a roan should not be crossed with a white-bellied hamster.

To determine if a black-eyed white is carrying the anophthalmic white gene, a light from a pen-torch can be shone in the eye. Carrier's eyes will glow ruby red in the centre. This test will also work for dark-eyed Dominant spots which may be carriers.

Cataracts

These may occur in older hamsters, and present as an opacity of the lens which is visible to the naked eye. They may also occur in association with diabetes. Because this is an inherited condition affected stock should not be used for breeding.

Affected hamsters may lose their sight completely, but are usually able to learn their surroundings and cope adequately as long as the furniture is not moved. Any levels in their cage from which they could fall should be removed.

THE EAR

Ear mites

Clinical signs: There are crusting lesions in the ears, and also on the face and feet. Infection is generally by the hamster ear mite *Notoedres notoedres* which is species specific, or the cat ear mite *Notoedres cati.*

Treatment: Ivermectin (Tx 13. Ivomec Injection for Cattle) can be given orally, or by subcutaneous injection.

THE MUSCULOSKELETAL SYSTEM

Limb fractures

These commonly occur from a fall, due either to being dropped, or falling in a tall cage. Hamsters can also catch their legs in open exercise wheels. Hamsters which eat a lot of sunflower seeds may have a subclinical calcium deficiency and therefore may be more susceptible to fractures.

Treatment: Immobilisation is difficult; the hamster is likely to chew at the dressing, leading to further complications. Closed fractures can be managed conservatively and although they may heal with abnormal angulation they do not hinder the hamster. The hamster should be kept in a solid sided tank for 6 weeks while healing is in progress. Fracture healing is fast with a callus forming within the first 7–10 days.

Open fractures may require limb amputation, which seems to be well tolerated.

Analgesia is important post-trauma with a non-steroidal anti-inflamatory drug.

Overgrown toenails

Older hamsters may need regular nail clipping, care being taken not to cut the quick. However, the blood vessels in the nail are small, so accidental blood loss should be minimal, and can be arrested with a suitable styptic.

Cage paralysis

Clinical signs: The affected hamster appears stiff and unable to move around, or moves around dragging its hind legs.

Treatment: As the disease is thought to be caused by lack of exercise, the hamster should be given a larger cage, and an exercise wheel provided. Vitamin supplementation may be beneficial, as it is thought that diets low in vitamins D and E predispose to the development of the condition (e.g. diets that are based on table scraps and are not balanced mixes).

Hind limb paralysis

Some male hamsters develop hind limb paralysis between 6 and 10 months of age. It is suggested this is a hereditary condition, associated with a sex-linked gene. Hamsters may also drag their hind legs in cage paralysis, constipation, dystocia or following spinal trauma.

MISCELLANEOUS CONDITIONS

Hibernation

This will occur if the environmental temperature drops below 5°C (41°F).

Clinical signs: Slow, shallow respiration and slow pulse. The hamster may appear dead.

Treatment: The hamster must be placed in a warm environment, on a heat-pad or hot-water bottle, or in the airing cupboard at a temperature of 30°C (86°F). Recovery may take up to an hour. The hamster will also recover if held gently in cupped hands for the same period, or upon gentle warming with a hair dryer. Once recovered the hamster can be given some glucose water from a dropper.

Comment: In the wild hamsters are not true hibernators, but if the day length shortens and the temperature falls they will gather food and pseudohibernate for extended periods. Pseudohibernation is most common in older animals, and may recur. Particular attention must be paid to the environment of affected animals.

Sleeper disease (heat stroke)

This occurs if the environmental temperature reaches 20–25°C (68–77°F).

Clinical signs: The hamster appears rigid and lifeless; it may rock its head from side to side. The fur may be wet and matted.

Treatment: Once cooled the hamster will soon return to normal. The recovered patient should be encouraged to drink.

Cases which have become particularly dehydrated may develop kidney failure. Fluid replacement is very important and oral rehydration solution (Tx 24. Lectade) is recommended for this purpose.

Lymphocytic chorio-meningitis virus (LCMV)

The natural hosts for this virus are wild mice, where the incidence of infection is nearly 100%. The infection can be transmitted to other rodents, and from hamsters to humans. It is spread in saliva, faeces, urine and milk. It is also spread by blood-sucking insect vectors, although the usual method of spread in hamsters is through bite wounds. In the wild mouse population LCMV can be transmitted *in utero*.

Clinical signs: In hamsters the disease is usually asymptomatic; an infected animal may develop a persistent tolerant infection for up to 6 months, during which time the virus is shed in the urine, faeces and saliva.

LCMV has been recorded as causing pyometra, poor reproductive performance, conjunctivitis and head tilt.

Comment: LCMV is a zoonosis, and hamsters and mice are considered to be the major source of infection for man. The disease in man resembles influenza, with fever, headache, rash, arthritis and rarely, fatal encephalomyelitis.

Hamster plague

This is caused by a virus, and little is known about the condition. Treatment is supportive with the provision of warmth and fluids.

Clinical signs: The hamster becomes cold, lethargic and dehydrated. It walks with its back arched and its eyes closed. Death usually occurs within 24 hours following a series of fits.

Diabetes

This is a relatively common condition of older hamsters. The main presenting sign is polydipsia, and subsequent polyuria. It is thought to be inherited in Russian and Chinese hamsters and affected individuals should not be used for breeding. Diabetic hamsters may live for several months after the diagnosis is made; they generally lose weight and may develop cataracts. Their frequent urination will require them to be given fresh, dry bedding daily.

12 ANAESTHESIA AND DRUG TREATMENTS

HANDLING

The hamster is best held in cupped hands, or scruffed for examination. It has a large scruff due to the size of the cheek pouches, and failure to grasp enough scruff will allow the hamster to turn and bite.

Care must be taken if the hamster is asleep in its nest as it is likely to bite if startled. Hamsters are very short-sighted and may bite in defence if they do not recognise the approaching hand. Chinese hamsters are the most docile.

NURSING

The prerequisites for good nursing are warmth, and comfortable clean surroundings. The environmental temperature should be between 23 and 25°C (73–77°F); this can be provided by a heat lamp, or by placing the cage in the airing cupboard. An aquarium makes a good hospital cage because it is well insulated.

PRE-ANAESTHETIC PREPARATION

Pre-anaesthetic starvation is unnecessary because regurgitation cannot occur due to the anatomy of the cardia of the stomach. Water should also remain available as any restriction can exaggerate the metabolic effects of anaesthesia.

The patient must be accurately weighed to enable drug doses to be correctly calculated. Because the hamster, in common with all small

139

rodents, has a small body size and high metabolic rate its potential to lose body heat and fluids during surgery is large. All small rodents are prone to hypothermia and circulatory shock when anaesthetised. These problems must be minimised by the following methods:

- The patient's body can be wrapped in aluminium foil or plastic bubble-wrap to conserve heat.
- The shaved surgical area should be the minimum size possible, and skin preparation done using warmed preparations. Care should be taken to avoid wetting the surrounding coat as this will lead to cooling by evaporation.
- If subcutaneous fluid therapy is given the solution must be warmed to the patient's body temperature.

PREMEDICATION

Atropine

Atropine should be given as a premedicant at a dose of 40 µg/kg by either subcutaneous or intramuscular injection to reduce salivation.

Dose: Atropine sulphate injection contains 600 µg/ml. An adult hamster weighing 115 g requires a dose of 0.007 ml subcutaneously. The atropine sulphate injection can be diluted 1:10 with sterile water for injection, providing a dose size of 0.07 ml.

ANAESTHESIA

Inhalation anaesthesia

Inhalation anaesthesia is the easiest method, using halothane, isoflurane or methoxyflurane with an oxygen/nitrous oxide combination. For induction a small see-through chamber can be constructed to allow the anaesthetic gas to enter, with holes which permit the gas to escape and be scavenged. The patient can remain in the chamber until the righting reflex is lost and then it can be transferred to and maintained on a face mask. Small face masks can be made with the ends of plastic syringe cases.

Halothane

Dose: The induction concentration of halothane should be 3–4%, and the maintenance concentration 1–2%.

Isoflurane

Dose: The induction concentration is 3.4–4.5%, and 1.5–3% is needed for maintenance.

Methoxyflurane

Dose: The induction concentration is 4%, with 0.4–1% for maintenance.

Ether

Ether is not recommended because it is highly irritant and explosive.

Injection anaesthesia

Injectable anaesthetics are available, and can be used. The size of the patient dictates that the injections are given subcutaneously, intramuscularly or intraperitoneally. Accurate dosing is essential.

Ketamine combinations can be used, and can be given by intraperitoneal injection.

Ketamine/acepromazine

Dose: 150 mg/kg ketamine plus 5 mg/kg acepromazine intraperitoneally.

Ketamine/xylazine

Dose: 200 mg/kg ketamine and 10 mg/kg xylazine by intraperitoneal injection.

Comment: Even when an injectable anaesthetic is used it is recommended that oxygen should be administered through the face mask during the operative procedure.

Anaesthetic monitoring

Monitoring the anaesthetic is not as easy as in a dog or cat because the hamster patient is much smaller. The most reliable indicator of surgical anaesthesia is the loss of withdrawal reflex in response to a painful stimulus such as a toe, tail or ear pinch. As the anaesthetic deepens the respiratory and cardiovascular parameters will be depressed.

Doxapram

Dopram (Willows Francis Ltd.)

This contains 20 mg/ml doxapram and is a useful respiratory stimulant.

Dose: 10 mg/kg can be given, i.e. 0.05 ml, by subcutaneous, intramuscular or intraperitoneal injection.

ANALGESIA

Analgesia is most effective if given before anaesthesia, or during the anaesthetic.

Buprenorphine

This is widely used.

Dose: 0.01–0.1 mg/kg subcutaneously every 6–12 hours.

After surgery non-steroidal analgesics can be given by mouth.

POST-OPERATIVE CARE

The hamster should be kept warm and quiet. Initially the external temperature should be 35°C (95°F), reducing to 25°C (77°F) once recovery is in progress. A heat-reflective surface, e.g. Flectabed, or vetbed is suitable; sawdust and shavings are not recommended as bedding because they will stick to wounds, and catch in the face and eyes.

Fluid replacement therapy

This is particularly valuable following surgery, or for any debilitated hamster.

Dose: 3 ml can be administered subcutaneously or via intraperitoneal injection. Glucose–saline (0.9% saline, 5% glucose) is the fluid of choice. The fluids should be warmed before administration.

INJECTION PROCEDURES

Subcutaneous injections can be made in the scruff of the neck, and up to 3–4 ml fluid can be given via this route.

Intramuscular injections can be given into the gluteal using a 25 gauge needle. The maximum volume that can be given in this site is 0.1 ml.

Intraperitoneal injections can be made with a 25 gauge needle. The hamster should be held on its back with one hind leg extended. The needle can be introduced along the line of this leg into the centre of the corresponding posterior quadrant of the abdomen and 2–3 ml of fluid can be given by this route.

Intravenous injections are very difficult because of the small size of the patient; the lateral tail vein is used for this procedure.

DRUG TREATMENTS

Because of their small size injections are best given by the subcutaneous, intraperitoneal, or intramuscular route. The patient should be weighed so that doses can be calculated correctly and an insulin syringe should be used for greatest accuracy.

The hamster's cheek pouches pose a problem when dosing orally, because the hamster may not take the required dose or may expel it from its cheek pouches after treatment.

Antibiotics

The administration of some antibiotics alters the intestinal microflora in a way which allows proliferation of *Clostridium* spp., particularly *Clostridium difficile*. This proliferation produces enterotoxins which cause fatal enteritis and diarrhoea. The most toxic drugs are those which have a narrow spectrum of activity against Gram-positive organisms, e.g. erythromycin, pencillin, lincomycin, cephalosporin and streptomycin.

Broad spectrum antibiotics are safer, and enrofloxacin, tetracycline, metronidazole and neomycin are recommended. When dosing with antibiotics it is important to give a probiotic and vitamin B concurrently, to protect against antibiotic-induced diarrhoea.

Tx 1. Enrofloxacin

Baytril (Bayer plc.)

Dose: 10 mg/kg daily
The 2.5% injection solution can be given subcutaneously at a dose of 0.02 ml/day. The 2.5% oral solution can be diluted 1:1 with blackcurrant syrup and given at a dose of 1 drop twice daily (dwarfs), or 2 drops twice daily (golden) by mouth. The dose can be soaked into a piece of puffed rice cereal to make dosing easier.

The oral 2.5% solution can be diluted to produce a drinking water concentration of 100 mg/litre by taking 4 ml and making it up to 1 litre with water.

Tx 2. Erythromycin

Erythrocin soluble (Sanfoni Animal Health)

This has been used as a preventative measure to control 'wet tail' in a colony situation.

Dose: The sachets contain 11.56 g erythromycin. One sachet diluted in 115 litres of water will provide a concentration of 100 mg/litre.

Tx 3. Metronidazole

Torgyl (Rhône Mérieux)

This contains 5 mg/ml metronidazole.

Dose: This can be given orally, especially in cases of 'wet tail' at a dose of 0.25 ml daily. Alternatively 20 ml can be diluted in 1 litre of water to produce a concentration of 100 mg/litre and used to replace the drinking water for 5–7 days.

Tx 4. Neomycin

Neobiotic Aquadrops (Upjohn Ltd.)

These contain 50 mg/ml neomycin which helps combat bacterial enteritis.

Dose: The drops can be diluted 1:3 with water and given at a dose of 1 drop twice daily. The maximum daily dose of neomycin is 10 mg (i.e. 0.1 ml undiluted aquadrops twice daily).

Tx 5. Oxytetracycline

Terramycin Soluble Powder 5.5% (Pfizer Ltd.)

This contains 55 g/kg oxytetracycline hydrochloride. A level scoopful approximately 4 g contains about 200 mg oxytetracycline.

Dose: One scoopful in 2 litres of drinking water gives a concentration of about 100 mg/litre; one scoopful in 0.5 litre gives a concentration of approximately 400 mg/litre.

Tx 6. Trimethoprim/sulphonamide

Borgal 7.5% (Hoechst UK Ltd.)

This contains 12.5 mg/ml trimethoprim and 62.5 mg/ml sulphadoxine.

Dose: This can be given by subcutaneous injection at a dose of 0.2 ml daily.

Probiotics

These can be given at the same time as antibiotics, or in times of dehabilitation, to improve the appetite.

Tx 7. Avipro (Vetark Health)

This is a water soluble probiotic, containing *Lactobacillus acidophilus*, *Enterococcus faecium*, *saccharomyces* and electrolytes.

Dose: It can be diluted in the drinking water at a rate of 5 g/200 ml water.

Comment: It is also useful in periods of stress, to protect the gastro-intestinal tract from stress-related disease.

Tx 8. Enterodex (Vydex Animal Health)

This contains the beneficial bacteria *Enterococcus*, similar to *Lactobacillus*.

Dose: One teaspoonful in the drinking water is sufficient for 40 hamsters. For single hamsters a small pinch can be mixed with the drinking water.

Antifungal agents

Tx 9. Griseofulvin

Grisovin tablets

The tablets each contain 125 mg griseofulvin.

Dose: The dose is 25 mg/kg. Assuming that not all the dry food is ingested one quarter of a tablet can be safely crushed and sprinkled on the dry food daily, for 3–4 weeks. Griseofulvin should not be given during pregnancy because it may be teratogenic.

Tx 10. Natamycin

Mycophyt (Mycofarm UK Ltd.)

This contains 1 g natamycin in 10 g.

Dose: 1 g of concentrate is mixed with 1 litre of water and used as a dip. It should not be rinsed off.

Tx 11. Povidone–iodine

Pevidine Antiseptic Solution (BK Veterinary Products)

Dose: This can be diluted 1:5 and used as a shampoo. Its effects are increased if the shampoo is left for 5 minutes before rinsing.

Ectoparasitic preparations

Tx 12. Amitraz

Aludex (Hoechst UK Ltd.)

This contains 50 g/litre amitraz.

Dose: The recommended concentration is 0.01% (100 ppm) amitraz; this is achieved by diluting 1 ml Aludex in 0.5 litre of water. The solution should be used as a dip, and not rinsed.

Tx 13. Ivermectin

Ivomec Injection for Cattle (Merck, Sharpe & Dohme Ltd.)

Ivomec contains 1% w/v ivermectin.

Dose: It can be given by subcutaneous injection at a dose rate of 200–400 µg/kg every 10 days. Ivomec can be diluted 1:10 with water and 0.02 ml given by injection.
   Alternatively, undiluted Ivomec can be given by mouth at a dose of 1 drop, repeated at 10 day intervals as necessary.
   Ivermectin can be used in conjunction with Aludex (Tx 12) baths.

Tx 14. Pyrethrin

Anti-mite Spray for Birds (Johnson)

This contains 0.8% w/v pyrethrin, and piperonyl butoxide BP.

Dose: A light spray may be given and repeated weekly if necessary.

Tx 15. Fipronil

Frontline (Rhône Mérieux)

This spray contains 0.25% w/v fipronil.

Dose: 7.5 mg/kg: it may be necessary to dilute with isopropyl alcohol to achieve this dose rate. The treatment may be repeated monthly.

Endoparasitic preparations

Tx 16. Piperazine

Antepar Elixir (Wellcome)

Antepar contains 150 mg/ml piperazine and will control nematodes (pinworms).

Dose: The required concentration of 2 mg/ml piperazine in the drinking water can be achieved by diluting the elixir 1:75 with water, and replacing the drinking water with this solution.

Tx 17. Nicolosamide

Troscan 100 (Bayer plc.)

These tablets each contain 100 mg niclosamide.

Dose: One tenth of a tablet can be given to an adult hamster, and the dose repeated after 7 days.

Miscellaneous treatments

Tx 18. Corticosteroids

These are useful in cases of both endotoxic shock, and shock following trauma.

Dexadreson (Intervet UK Ltd.)

This contains a rapid action formulation of dexamethasone at a concentration of 2 mg/ml.

Dose: Dexadreson can be given by intramuscular injection at a dose of 0.01–0.02 ml.

Tx 19. Kaolin/pectin mixture

Kaogel (Parke Davis & Co Ltd.)

Kaogel contains 20% w/v light kaolin, and 0.43% w/v pectin. Many paediatric diarrhoea preparations are similar, and make suitable alternatives.

Dose: 0.1–0.2 ml (two or three drops) orally three times daily, as an adjunct to other diarrhoea therapy.

Tx 20. Pseudoephedrine hydrochloride

Sudafed (Wellcome)

This contains 6 mg/ml pseudoephedrine hydrochloride.

Dose: One drop can be given twice daily.

Tx 21. Dermisol (Pfizer Ltd.)

This is a topical preparation which contains propylene glycol, malic acid, benzoic acid and salicylic acid. It promotes healing by removing dead and necrotic tissue from affected areas and also has antibacterial properties. It can be applied two or three times daily.

Tx 22. Lactated Ringer's solution (Hartmann's solution)

This contains 3.1 g sodium lactate, 6 g sodium chloride, 0.4 g potassium chloride and 0.7 g calcium chloride per litre.

Dose: The maximum amount for fluid replacement is 3 ml by subcutaneous or intraperitoneal injection.

Tx 23. Glucose–saline

5% glucose with 0.9% saline.

Dose: The maximum amount for fluid replacement is 3 ml by subcutaneous or intraperitoneal injection.

Tx 24. Oral rehydration solution

Lectade (Pfizer Ltd.)

Lectade is an oral rehydration solution containing dextrose monohydrate, sodium chloride, aminoacetic acid, potassium citrate and citric acid.

Dose: The liquid form can be diluted 20 ml lectade into 250 ml water, and given orally whenever fluid replacement is indicated.

Tx 25. Lactulose

Duphalac (Solvay Healthcare)

This contains 3.35 g lactulose in 5 ml.

Dose: One or two drops may be given twice daily.

Eye preparations

Tx 26. Chloromycetin Ophthalmic Ointment 1% (Parke, Davis & Co. Ltd.)

This contains chloramphenicol and can be applied twice daily, or more frequently if required, for 5 days.

Tx 27. Neobiotic HC (Upjohn Ltd.)

This contains the antibiotic neomycin and hydrocortisone as the steroid. It is a ready flowing liquid and can be applied two or three times daily.

Tx 28. Maxitrol (Alcon Ltd.)

This contains an antibiotic (neomycin), steroid (dexamethasone), and an antifungal agent (polymyxin B). It can be applied two or three times daily.

Tx 29. Golden Eye Ointment (Typharm Ltd.)

This is available from pharmacists and contains dibromopropamidine isethionate 0.15 w/w and liquid paraffin. It is useful for minor eye infections and conjunctivitis. It can be applied once or twice daily.

MICE

The mice most commonly kept as pets today are *Mus musculus*. Mice have been associated with humans for thousands of years, and were worshipped in some religions as long as 4000 years ago.

Mice are available in white, self (solid body colour) in a variety of colours, or marked with white and a specific pattern of coloured patches, e.g. Dutch or Himalayan.

'Waltzing' mice are a mutation resulting from a recessive gene which causes growth retardation and middle ear damage which leads to deafness and incoordination, the latter giving rise to their name as they spin around in circles.

13 HUSBANDRY AND NUTRITION

Environment

Where only a few mice are owned they can be kept indoors. The room temperature should be between 15 and 27°C (59–80°F) (18–22°C (64–72°F) is best). Temperatures over 30°C (86°F) may cause heatstroke. Good lighting is important, but no cages should be placed in direct sunlight as they will quickly heat up. The relative humidity should be between 40 and 70%; over 50% is optimal.

Larger numbers of mice are best kept outdoors, in a shed or out-building. Mice can withstand colder temperatures as long as they have plenty of bedding. If they are kept outside it is very important to prevent the entry of wild rodents which may be carriers of disease.

Good ventilation is important; however, any windows should be protected by mesh to prevent the entry of predators, especially cats.

Housing

A wide variety of accommodation can be provided for mice, but the general principles are the same. The cage must be well ventilated, easy to clean, and escape-proof. Many cages have gaps in the bars which may be large enough for a small mouse to crawl through. Cages can be made out of plastic or wood, with wire tops or sides for ventilation; glass aquariums can also be used. Wood will soak up the urine; it will therefore smell and be harder to keep clean. Mice are active gnawers and this must be taken into consideration.

The recommended cage size is 45 cm × 45 cm × 23 cm (l × w × h), although the larger the cage the better. Inside the cage furnishings can include a nest-box, an exercise wheel and other toys such as tubes and jars.

Cardboard tubes can be used; however, the cardboard has a short life-span because it is likely to be chewed and will soak up urine.

Bedding

The bedding and floor litter should be absorbent. Sawdust is excellent floor covering and shoud be 1 cm deep. It should be bought in special packed bales, and not as floor sweepings from the local sawmill because the latter may be contaminated with urine from wild rodents and thus carry disease. Good quality hay should be provided on top. To minimise odours a little baking soda (sodium carbonate) can be sprinkled in the corners of the cage. Shredded unprinted paper can also be used for bedding; care must be taken with synthetic bedding because it may cause impactions if ingested.

The bedding and floor litter should be changed weekly, because the ammonia from urine can build up and predispose to mycoplasmal respiratory infections; soiled corners may need changing more frequently.

Stocking

For breeding purposes mice can be kept in a monogamous or polygamous (harem) system. Pet mice not kept for breeding are happiest kept in pairs, and a pair of males, or a pair of females may live together. Females tend to be more docile, and less likely to fight. Females also give off less odour, an important consideration if they are to be kept as pets indoors.

Nutrition

For their staple diet in the wild, mice feed on starch-filled seeds, especially grains, rice and millet. In captivity they could, given the opportunity, eat most foodstuffs, but they may select foods that are bad for them.

A basic staple diet for mice can be oats and bread. Commercially produced rations are also available and these can be supplemented with small amounts of fruit, vegetables and dog biscuits. The last are excellent for gnawing and promoting an even wear on the teeth.

All food should be provided in solid containers that cannot be easily chewed, tipped over or soiled. Fresh water from a sipper bottle should be available at all times. The average water intake is 4 ml daily for an adult mouse.

Mice become accustomed to a daily routine, and are best fed at the same time each day.

Carbohydrates

Oats can be fed whole or crushed. They should not be dusty because this may trigger respiratory disease. A tablespoonful of oats daily should be adequate for an adult mouse.

Bread can be either white or brown; however, the latter is preferable. It should be stale and hard, or baked in an oven to dry it. It can be fed hard, which will encourage gnawing, or it can then be soaked in water to moisten it (excess moisture should be squeezed out so that it is not sloppy). Milk can be added to the bread mixture; this is particularly useful for lactating females.

Other grains can be fed, but a proprietary grain mix for rodents (e.g. hamsters) should be used with caution. The mice may selectively pick out a particular seed which may be harmful if eaten in excess. Too many sunflower seeds, wheat or maize lead to overheating, and pruritic skin lesions. Canary or budgie seed can be given occasionally.

Dog biscuits can be provided and are useful for gnawing.

Fresh food

A small variety of fresh food helps make the diet interesting, and provides additional minerals and vitamins. Any fresh food should be introduced slowly and in small amounts to prevent scouring. Root vegetables such as carrot and swede are suitable, and greens such as celery, cabbage and cauliflower leaves can be offered. Wild plants that can be given are shepherd's purse (astringent), and dandelion and groundsel (both laxative).

Hay

Good quality hay should be used for the bedding material, and it will be eaten by the mice providing fibre for the digestive system. The hay should not be dusty or mouldy which would predispose to respiratory disease.

Vitamins

If a balanced diet is fed, vitamin supplementation should not be necessary.

The most important vitamins are A and D. These can be found in cod-liver oil, and this can be added to the bread mix. Vitamin E is present in wheatgerm, and is useful in cases of apparent infertility. Linseed oil can be given as a supplement to improve coat condition.

14   SYSTEMS AND DISEASES

THE SKIN

Diet-associated dermatitis

Many of the skin lesions seen in pet mice are associated with the feeding of an incorrect diet. These mice are often fed a proprietary rodent or hamster mix which is full of nuts and sunflower seeds containing oils and fats which, in excessive quantities, can trigger intensely pruritic skin lesions. Such mixes may also contain pieces of coloured biscuit, with dyes that may cause an allergic dermatitis.

Clinical signs: These include intense pruritus, wet dermatitis and self-excoriation which may lead to lesions bleeding around the head and neck.

Treatment: All previous food should be withdrawn, and a simpler diet of oats and bread should be fed. Once the symptoms are resolved additional foods can be added to the diet on a trial basis, and any which cause pruritus should be removed. A corticosteroid injection (Tx 14 or 15) can be given to relieve the pruritus in the initial stages of treatment.

Ringworm

This is not common in mice, but some may carry unapparent infections.

Clinical signs: There are small scaly lesions, and some alopecia.

Diagnosis: Microscopy and culture on Sabouraud's medium are necessary. If the ringworm is caused by *Microsporum* spp. the lesions will fluoresce under ultraviolet light.

Treatment: Griseofulvin (Tx 16) can be given in the food for 4–6

157

weeks. Enilconazole (Tx 17. Imaverol) can be made up to a 10% solution and used as a weekly dip.

Fleas

These are rare, but may be *Ctenocephalides felis* caught from an in-contact dog or cat. They are visible to the naked eye.

Treatment: A spray containing pyrethrin is safe to use, or a pyrethrin powder. Dichlorvos strips, e.g. Vapona, can be placed in the room or shed and this will help repel flies and ectoparasites. The cage must also be thoroughly cleaned and sprayed with a pyrethrin spray (Tx 11. Anti-mite Spray for Birds). The bedding and floor litter should be changed.

Lice and mites

These are rare in pet mice, they are generally brought in via bedding or materials that have been contaminated by wild mice, or through the movement of infected stock. Mice are affected by the louse *Polyplax serrata*, and the mites *Myobia musculi* and *Myocoptes musculinus*.

Sarcoptic mange caused by *Sarcoptes scabiei* is rare; demodectic mange caused by *Demodex creceti* may be seen if the mouse is immunosuppressed or has concurrent debilitating disease.

Clinical signs: Ulcerating lesions on the back are caused by mites. Clusters of ectoparasites may occur around the neck and ears leading to pruritus in these areas. The fur may become greasy. The parasite can be identified by microscopy.

Treatment: Dusting with pyrethrin powder. Diluted fipronil (Tx 10. Frontline) at a concentration of 7.5 mg/kg can be applied. In the case of sarcoptic or demodectic mange Ivermectin (Tx 9) can be given orally, or amitraz (Tx 8) can be used as a dip in a 0.01% solution.

Dichlorvos strips, e.g. Vapona, hung outside the cage will reduce the ectoparasite population. The cage should be cleaned, and can be sprayed with a pyrethrin spray (Tx 11). The bedding should be replaced.

Barbering

Dominant members of a group may barber the other mice. The hair is chewed short down to the skin, and often the whiskers are completely chewed. The hair loss is often bilateral. The dominant mouse in the group will be the one that is not chewed. The dominant mouse may need to be removed and more space created for the group of mice in order to prevent boredom and bullying. Whisker biting may be hereditary, and mice with this trait should not be bred from.

Alopecia

Hair loss may be associated with barbering, or the ectoparasites mentioned previously. Hormonal alopecia is also recognised; the hair loss is usually symmetrical over each flank. Abrasions on feeders, or rubbing on the cage bars may lead to facial alopecia.

Bite wounds and abscesses

Bites usually occur on the tail and rump. Male mice should not be housed together because fighting is likely. In a group situation the dominant mouse may need to be removed. Stresses such as overcrowding must be avoided.

Subcutaneous abscesses may also occur as a result of bacterial infection, usually by *Actinobacillus* or *Corynebacterium* spp. An ulcerative dermatitis may be caused by *Staphylococcus aureus*.

Treatment: Wounds should be cleaned with a mild antiseptic or saline solution, and antibiotics (Tx 1–6) given systemically or orally. An antiseptic powder, e.g. Ster-zac, can be used on the wound.

Abscesses and ulcerative dermatitis must be treated with oral or systemic antibiotics (Tx 1–6).

Neoplasia

Tumours of the skin are rare, although neoplasia of the mammary glands is common and frequently malignant. Squamous cell carcinomas are seen infrequently. Surgical removal of tumours is not advisable due to the high potential for recurrence and metastasis. The affected mouse may be able to live with its growth for some time before euthanasia is indicated.

Mousepox (ectromelia virus)

Mousepox is seen in laboratory mice.

Clinical signs: These are variable and range from papules and crusting around the face to necrosis of the extremities of the limbs and tail.

Diagnosis: This is based on the clinical signs and histopathology.

Comment: The virus is very contagious to other mice, and the scabs and debris are also infective. Affected mice should be culled, the bedding and floor litter destroyed, and the environment thoroughly disinfected.

THE REPRODUCTIVE SYSTEM

- Litter size: 8–12
- Birth weight: 1–2 g
- Weaning age: 3–4 weeks
- Puberty: 6–7 weeks
- Oestrus cycle: 4–5 days
- Post partum oestrus: fertile
- Duration of oestrus: 12 hours
- Gestation: 19–21 days

Sexing

Male mice have a greater anogenital distance, up to twice as long as the female (Figure 14.1). In the young male the testes may be visible through the abdominal wall. From the age of 9 days females have a visible set of two rows of nipples.

Breeding

Mice can be bred in a monogamous or polygamous (harem) system. A monogamous system will allow the male to be removed before parturition to prevent a post-partum mating. A polygamous system may make identification of the dam of the litter difficult, and females may cannibalise young that are not their own.

Breeding stock should be given plenty of nesting material, and a nest box made of wood or cardboard for security.

Oestrus

Mice are polyoestrous and come into season all year round. In a group situation female mice may come into oestrus together, this synchronisation

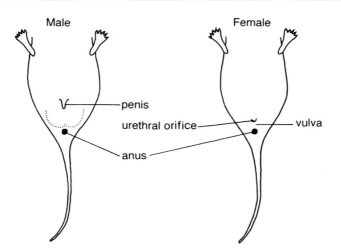

Figure 14.1 External genitalia.

is known as the Whitten effect. The oestrus cycle is 4–6 days long, and oestrus lasts 12 hours, generally from early evening and overnight. The length of the oestrus cycle increases with age. The oestrus cycle also lengthens in the absence of a male. A post-partum oestrus occurs 12 hours after parturition and a mating at this time will be fertile. Oestrus does not occur during lactation. The subsequent oestrus occurs 2–5 days after weaning.

Mating

Although mice are capable of breeding at 6 weeks of age they should not be first mated until they are 11–12 weeks old and have attained a weight of 20–30 g. Mating generally takes place in the late evening. After mating a copulatory plug from secretions from the male accessory glands is formed, and this remains in the vulva for 24–48 hours before dropping out.

Pseudopregnancy

This can occur following a sterile mating. It may last between 1 and 3 weeks after which the doe returns to oestrus. Pseudopregnancy can also occur in the absence of a male; in this instance exposure to a male or the smell of his urine will cause the doe to return to oestrus in 2–3 days.

Gestation

Gestation lasts for 19–21 days. If the pregnancy is a result of a post-partum mating and the doe is lactating, delayed implantation may occur lengthening the apparent gestation period by 3–10 days. Pregnancy can be detected by a noticeable weight gain from day 13 of gestation. Mammary development increases in the third week of gestation.

Parturition

Before parturition the doe begins avid nest building. Often mice that have had plenty of time and materials to make a good nest make the best mothers. A few hours before delivery commences a vaginal discharge may be evident, and the doe may make repeated stretching movements. Parturition generally takes place at night and lasts 30 minutes. The doe must not be disturbed at this time or she may abandon or cannibalise her litter. The young are born naked and blind, and weigh 1–2 gm each. Any young born dead will usually be eaten by the doe.

Development of the young

At birth the young are naked and blind with closed ears. The ears open at 4 days, and the young are fully haired in 7–10 days. The eyes open on days 12–14 and the incisors erupt between days 11 and 13. The young should be sexed, separated and weaned between 21 and 25 days of age.

Dystocia

This may occur if the foeti are especially large or malpresented.

Clinical signs: The female fails to produce a litter after the 21 days gestation, and may develop a stary coat, diarrhoea and a vaginal discharge.

Treatment: Intervention is difficult due to patient size, although Caesarean section could be attempted. An old remedy is to give a few drops of liquid paraffin or castor oil with the wet food.

Uterine prolapse

This is rare, but may occur after a difficult birth or abortion.

Treatment: Replacement can be attempted but the prognosis is poor if the uterus re-prolapses.

Cannibalism

The doe must be left undisturbed for at least 2 days and preferably longer after parturition otherwise she may abandon or cannibalise her young.

Other reasons why a doe may desert her litter are if she is under-nourished and has agalactia or concurrent disease. If there is little nesting material and little privacy the doe may abandon her young. External disturbances such as high pitched sounds are another trigger factor.

Mastitis

This is not common in mice. It may be associated with poor husbandry and sanitation.

Clinical signs: One gland or more may become swollen, warm and painful. Needle aspiration will reveal purulent material, and help differentiate the condition from mammary gland neoplasia which is more common.

Treatment: The gland should be lanced, drained and cleaned. Antibiotics (Tx 1–6) can be given orally or systemically and recovery is usually good.

Mammary gland neoplasia

This is very common in mice from the age of 1 year. Some strains may have a familial predisposition to tumour development. The tumours are often spontaneous and malignant adenocarcinomas. Metastasis to the lungs is a frequent sequel.

Treatment: Surgery may be attempted but the prognosis is usually poor due to the malignant nature of the growths. Mice are able to accommodate fairly large growths and euthanasia need only be considered when the mouse becomes bothered by the growth.

Problems with the male

Testicular tumours

Tumours of the interstitial cells of the testes have been recorded, and castration carries a good prognosis because they have a low metastasis potential.

Clinical signs: A testicular tumour presents as a hard swelling in the testicle; the opposite testicle may shrink.

Treatment: The inguinal canals remain open throughout life. For castration a scrotal incision can be made to remove the testes, and the vas deferens and spermatic cord blood vessels ligated. The tunic and skin may be closed together as a single layer. The remaining adipose tissue appears to block the inguinal canals and prevent herniation.

Infertility

- In the female the litter size starts to decrease from 6–7 months of age and breeding may naturally stop between $1-1\frac{1}{2}$ years of age.
- If a large number of does are kept together without the presence of a male, their cycle length will increase and they may enter anoestrus. A few does kept together without a male may exhibit pseudopregnancy. The presence of a male, or the smell of his urine, should return these groups of females to oestrus.
- Photoperiod influences the breeding cycle, and a 12 hours darkness/12 hours light cycle is recommended. The light provided should be shaded natural light or artificial light, not direct sunlight.
- Low environmental temperature may inhibit breeding.
- External noise, and the presence of smells of chemicals or other predators may prevent breeding.
- Exposure to organophosphate compounds may cause infertility.
- If a mouse that has been mated is exposed to a strange male with 24 hours post-mating the litter may be aborted, leading to apparent infertility.
- Infertility may result following infection with *Pasteurella pneumotropica*, *Mycoplasma pulmonis*, *Klebsiella*, or *Streptobacillus moniliformis*.
- A vitamin E deficiency will lead to poor reproductive performance, smaller weak litters and young born with hind limb paralysis. Vitamin E

can be added to the food by incorporating wheatgerm or wheatgerm oil into the daily mix or bread mixture.

THE DIGESTIVE SYSTEM

Malocclusion

Occasionally the incisor teeth may not wear evenly, grow long and need subsequent trimming. The mouse will have difficulty eating and lose weight. Salivation is not usually a symptom. The mouse should be provided with plenty of foods to gnaw on; dog biscuits are suitable for this, or hard baked bread. The teeth should be checked regularly as the condition is likely to recur.

Diarrhoea

Diarrhoea in young stock is common and may be associated with endo-parasites, coccidiosis, bacterial disease or sudden dietary change. Adults contract diarrhoea less frequently, and parasites or diet are the most common causal agents. Severe diarrhoea can be devastating, and losses high. Strict hygiene is important to prevent the spread of any contagious problem. For milder cases all that may be necessary is to stop any wet or green food, and feed dry bread, and arrowroot biscuits or powder. Corn-flour can also be given.

Following are five specific causes of diarrhoea.

Protozoa and coccidia

Faecal examination may reveal the protozoa *Entamoeba muris*, *Trichomonas muris* and *Giardia muris*; in small numbers these are non-pathogenic. Small numbers of the coccidia *Eimeria* may also be found. However in conditions of poor husbandry, or concurrent disease, protozoa and coccidia can build up into large numbers and become pathogenic.

Clinical signs: Protozoa may cause a mild enteritis; coccidia may cause a range of symptoms ranging from a mild diarrhoea, to severe haemorrhagic and mucoid diarrhoea with a foul smell, colicky pains, a hunched up appearance and weight loss.

Treatment: Protozoal infections can be treated with metronidazole (Tx 19) in the drinking water at a rate of 2.5 mg/ml.

Coccidia can be treated with sulphadimidine (Tx 5. Intradine) in the drinking water for 7–10 days. The bedding must be kept as clean and dry as possible because coccidia thrive in damp surroundings. Mice can be given rabbit pellets containing a coccidiostat to try and control the infection; these should be introduced slowly into the daily diet.

Tapeworms and roundworms

Mice can be infected with the dwarf tapeworm *Hymenolepis nana*.

Clinical signs: Infected adult mice rarely show clinical signs, but heavy burdens in young mice may lead to symptoms of weight loss, diarrhoea and even intestinal obstruction.

Diagnosis: The eggs can be identified by faecal examination.

Treatment: Niclosamide (Tx 12. Troscan 100) is effective; one thirtieth of a tablet may be given to an adult mouse and the dose repeated after 7 days.

Control is difficult because this tapeworm has both an indirect life cycle through insect vectors and a direct life cycle which leads to autoinfection. Although the use of dichlorvos (e.g. Vapona) sticky strips will reduce the insect vectors, autoinfection cannot be prevented.

The pinworm *Syphacia obvelata* may be non-pathogenic in small numbers. It has a direct life cycle; the eggs are laid on the perineal skin and reingested by the affected mouse.

Clinical signs: Heavy burdens in younger animals may lead to diarrhoea and failure to thrive.

Diagnosis: The eggs can be collected with sticky tape and examined by microscopy to confirm the diagnosis.

Treatment: Ivermectin (Tx 9. Ivomec) is effective. Piperazine (Tx 13. Antepar) can also be used.

Bacteria

Clinical signs: Diarrhoea may be caused by several bacterial infections, and the clinical signs may be similar, including diarrhoea, loss of condition, rectal prolapse and occasional sudden death. When a large population of mice is at risk from a contagious bacterial infection it may be necessary to consider culling affected animals to prevent the disease spreading through the stock. If small numbers are involved treatment can be implemented.

Bacterial agents are *Salmonella typhimurium*, *Citrobacter freundii* and *Clostridium piliforme* (Tyzzer's disease). However, if the normal bacteria in the gut are allowed to proliferate they may also cause diarrhoea.

Diagnosis: Differential diagnosis of these bacteria can be done by faecal culture, or histological examination at necropsy. *Citrobacter freundii* causes a colonic mucosal hyperplasia, Tyzzer's disease produces characteristic white foci in the liver, *Salmonella typhimurium* produces a septicaemia with necrotic foci in liver and spleen. Rectal prolapse is most common with *Citrobacter freundii*.

Treatment: If treatment is undertaken antibiotics (Tx 1–6) should be given via the drinking water. Affected individuals should be put on a dry diet of oats, and arrowroot can be given in powder or biscuit form. Burnt toast can be offered and is beneficial. Strict hygiene and cage cleaning is essential to prevent the spread of infection.

Viruses

Viruses that may cause diarrhoea in mice are rotavirus, reovirus or coronavirus. The diarrhoea is often yellow and sticky, and affects unweaned mice.

Dietary

A sudden change of diet, the feeding of too much wet and green food, or mouldy hay or greens may lead to scouring.

Clinical signs: The affected mouse may still appear well and continue to eat.

Treatment: All wet food should be stopped; the mouse can be fed hay and dry oats. Arrowroot powder or arrowroot biscuits are also astringent. A few drops of a kaolin/pectin mixture (Tx 18) can be given orally two or three times daily.

THE RESPIRATORY SYSTEM

Respiratory disease is relatively common. It may be acute or chronic, and if an infection it is often a mixed infection. Respiratory disease may be triggered by stress, overcrowding, dusty bedding or the build up of damp bedding and thus ammonia from the urine. Breeders recognise symptoms of respiratory disease and refer to them as 'asthma', although they may be infectious or allergic in origin. Certain strains of mice may be prone to developing this problem, and selective breeding may help reduce the incidence of these 'asthma' symptoms. Clinical signs vary from wheezing, a rapid 'clicking' sound as the mouse breathes, dyspnoea, loss of appetite and lethargy. If a lot of mice are at risk it may be better to cull the affected individual to prevent the spread of disease; however, if only a few mice are involved treatment can be undertaken.

Allergic disease

Mice may be allergic to components of their bedding, fine sawdust or dusty hay. To test this theory they can be bedded on shredded white paper or kitchen towel. If kept indoors they may be sensitive to cigarette smoke, and aerosols such as furniture polish.

Clinical signs: These include rhinitis, sneezing and conjunctivitis. The affected mouse remains active and continues to eat and drink normally. Often only one of a group is affected, although certain strains of mice may be more prone to developing allergies than others.

Respiratory infections

Infection may be caused by *Pasteurella pneumotropica*, *Klebsiella pneumoniae*, *Bordetella bronchiseptica*, *Mycoplasma pulmonis*, Sendai virus, and pneumonia virus of mice, amongst others. Infections are often mixed, and may produce upper respiratory or lower respiratory tract symptoms or both.

Clinical signs: In response to stress the Harderian glands in the eye produce 'red tears', and there is porphyrin staining around the eyes and nose. Upper respiratory tract symptoms are sneezing and face-rubbing. Lower respiratory tract symptoms present with wheezing, dyspnoea, anorexia, weight loss and lethargy and a hunched-up posture.

Four respiratory infections will be described in more detail.

Mycoplasmosis

Mycoplasma pulmonis is carried sub-clinically in the upper respiratory tract and causes disease if the respiratory epithelium is weakened by other factors, such as stress, the build up of ammonia, or bacterial infection.

Clinical signs: These include rhinitis and nasal discharge. Otitis interna may present as torticollis.

   If the mycoplasmal infection is complicated by bacteria, or triggered by excess ammonia, lower respiratory tract symptoms will be evident too. These present as lethargy, hunched posture, dyspnoea and weight loss.

   A third presentation involves urogenital symptoms, infertility, resorption of litters and endometritis.

Treatment: Treatment may eliminate the clinical signs, but will not remove the carrier state. Improvements in cage sanitation and the avoidance of ammonia build up may prevent further outbreaks in infected stock. Oxytetracycline (Tx 6) can be given via the drinking water.

Pseudotuberculosis

Clinical signs: Infection with *Corynebacterium kutscheri* may be sub-clinical, or symptoms may reflect the abscesses caused in the lungs and abdominal organs by this bacterium, when a chronic debilitating weight loss is seen.

Treatments: Antibiotics (Tx 1–6) may limit the clinical signs, but the disease may continue to spread through sub-clinical carriers of the organism.

Sendai virus infection

Sendai virus is a paramyxovirus, which may not cause disease on its own, but may cause respiratory symptoms if mycoplasma are also present. In an enzootic situation the young mice receive passive immunity from their mothers for the first 6–8 weeks of life.

Mouse hepatitis virus infection

This virus initially affects the nasal passages; it may then spread to the intestines alone, or progress to a respiratory tract infection and spread to other organs in the body.

Clinical signs: The most serious symptoms appear in the young; a hunched posture, ruffled coat, diarrhoea and death. Adults usually exhibit mild symptoms and recover in 7–10 days. In an enzootic situation the young are protected by maternal antibodies when they are most vunerable to infection and symptoms are less severe.

Treatment: Adults need supportive nursing only whilst they are recovering.

Supportive treatment for respiratory disease

If only one or more mice are affected and treatment is instigated, antibiotics should be given where indicated. Because many respiratory infections are mixed, and often secondary bacterial infection is present, antibiotics (Tx 1–6) should be given orally or systemically. The affected individuals should be housed in a warm and clean environment, without compromising good ventilation. Mentholated ointment (e.g. Vick) can be smeared around the cage to help clear the nasal passages. A multivitamin solution containing vitamins A, C, D and B complex can be given (Tx 22. Abidec); one drop daily is sufficient for an average mouse.

THE EYE

The Harderian glands

These glands are in the medial canthus of the eye and they produce a red-brown secretion. This secretion is made up of porphyrins which give it its colour, and it should not be confused with blood. The secretions increase in situations of stress; concurrent disease and red crusting will be seen around the eyes and nose. These 'red tears' may appear associated with respiratory infection, but they may also occur in the absence of any respiratory involvement. Neoplasia of these glands may also occur.

Treatment: Any stress factors should be eliminated, and antibiotics given if there is concurrent disease. If the eyes are sore they should be gently bathed with mild saline solution (5 g salt dissolved in 500 ml water), and an eye ointment containing tetracycline or chlortetracycline (Tx 25. Aureomycin Ophthalmic Ointment) is recommended.

THE EAR

Middle ear disease

This is usually associated with a bacterial or mycoplasmal infection.

Clinical signs: Circling, head tilt, loss of balance. At post-mortem the middle ear is found to be full of pus and debris.

Treatment: Antibiotics (Tx 1–6) may relieve the clinical signs, although in some cases they may be required for long periods. There may only be a partial resolution of the symptoms, but a pet mouse may be able to compensate adequately.

Defective middle ear

Circling and loss of balance is seen in 'waltzing' mice. This is an inherited condition; the gene responsible produces a defect in the middle ear. These mice are often spotted black and white, and have stunted growth. Such mice should not be bred from.

Otitis externa

Mice may be infected with the ear mite *Notoedres muris*. Clinical signs include pruritus and wax build up in the ear. Ivermectin (Tx 9) is effective and can be given orally or by subcutaneous injection.

Sores around the ears and scratching around the head and neck may also be a symptom of food allergy. If no signs of ear or fur mites are present a plain diet should be tried (see Skin section).

THE MUSCULOSKELETAL SYSTEM

Paralysis

Posterior paralysis most commonly occurs as a result of spinal trauma following a fall, but rarely may occur as a result of viral infection. Lymphocytic choriomeningitis virus (LCMV) may be asymptomatic in mice, but may result in paralysis and death. Mouse encephalomyelitis virus is also extremely rare; symptoms are general malaise and progressive posterior paralysis as a result of poliomyelitis and demyelination. Mice showing neurological symptoms should be culled because of the potential zoonotic risk of these viruses. LCMV causes influenza-like symptoms in people, and although rare it must be considered in their differential diagnosis.

Fractures

Limb fractures are usually the result of a traumatic injury or a fall. Unstable fractures can be taped with a stretch fabric plaster, e.g. Elastoplast; however, the mouse may chew at the dressing and traumatise the fracture further. Stable fractures will heal without dressing, provided the mouse is kept in a small cage with no opportunity to climb or jump; a plastic bowl or aquarium is suitable for this. A callus forms at the fracture site in as little as 7–10 days.

Kinked tails

Mice born with kinked tails should not be bred from because the condition is inherited. Kinked tails may also be acquired in later life as a result of a traumatic injury, but should heal without intervention. The only exception is if the tail becomes degloved at the time of the injury; if this is the case the damaged tail may require amputation under general anaesthetic.

Pododermatitis

This may occur if environmental conditions are poor, if the mice are housed on rough or wire floors with little floor litter and bedding, or if these become very soiled. Obese animals may be most prone to developing lesions.

Clinical signs: One or more feet may become swollen or ulcerated, and the infection may ascend up the affected leg and cause distal joint swelling.

Treatment: The affected animal should be moved onto dry soft bedding. The lesions can be bathed in a mild saline solution (5 g salt dissolved in 500 ml water), and antibiotics (Tx 1–6) should be given orally or systemically.

Antibiotic or antiseptic creams can be applied topically. Sudocrem (Tx 23) or Dermisol (Tx 24) are suitable.

Osteoarthritis

This is fairly common in older mice, and may cause a stiffness and reluctance to move. Mice can be given non-steroidal anti-inflammatory drugs such as aspirin (Tx 20) or paracetamol (Tx 21) (see also Analgesia in Chapter 15). The dose of aspirin for a 30 g mouse is 3.6 mg (120 mg/kg). Soluble aspirin could be given in the drinking water at a concentration of 1 mg/ml.

MISCELLANEOUS CONDITIONS

Leptospirosis

Leptospira spp. are important as they have zoonotic potential. Clinical infection in mice is rare, but wild mice are considered to be the natural reservoir of this bacteria, and pet mice could contract infection if their food, bedding or environment has been soiled by wild mice. Pet mice may become symptomless carriers; the leptospires are harboured in the kidneys and shed in the urine.

Human infection may result in vague malaise or influenza-like symptoms, with fever, headache, myalgia, conjunctivitis and skin rashes. Although leptospirosis is rare it must be considered as a diagnosis in any person that keeps rodents and has such symptoms.

Affected animals should be culled because of the public health implications.

Hypothermia

Because the mouse has a high metabolic rate it relies on a ready source of food, and adequate bedding so that it can maintain its body temperature. If the mouse has scant bedding and small food reserves it is at risk from hypothermia.

Clinical signs: Affected mice may appear weak or comatose. The extremities will feel chilled.

Treatment: Gentle warming may resolve the condition. The mouse can be placed in cupped hands, or close to a heat source, such as by a lamp bulb or in the airing cupboard. It should not be placed directly on a heat source as this will cause vasodilation and may lead to shock. The mouse should be encouraged to eat or drink, and if necessary can be given warmed water containing a little glucose or sugar by syringe.

15 ANAESTHESIA AND DRUG TREATMENTS

HANDLING

Mice can be picked up gently by the base of the tail, and then steadied by the scruff of the neck with the thumb and fore-finger. The grip on the tail can be transferred to the third and fourth finger so that the mouse is lying across the palm of the hand.

PRE-ANAESTHETIC PREPARATION

Pre-anaesthetic starvation is unnecessary as mice are unable to vomit. Water should also be made available right up until the induction of anaesthesia, as dehydration may potentiate the anaesthetic effects.

The patient must be accurately weighed to enable drug doses to be correctly calculated. Because the mouse, in common with all small rodents, has a small body size and high metabolic rate its potential to lose body heat and fluids during surgery is large. All small rodents are prone to hypothermia and circulatory shock when anaesthetised. These problems must be minimised by the following methods:

- The patient's body can be wrapped in aluminium foil or plastic bubble-wrap to conserve heat.
- The shaved surgical area should be the minimum size possible, and skin preparation done using warmed preparations. Care should be taken to avoid wetting the surrounding coat as this will lead to cooling by evaporation.
- If subcutaneous fluid therapy is given the solution must be warmed to the patient's body temperature.

PREMEDICATION

Atropine

Atropine should be given as a premedicant at a dose of 40 μg/kg by either subcutaneous or intramuscular injection to reduce salivation.

Dose: Atropine sulphate injection contains 600 μg/ml. An adult mouse weighing 30 g requires a dose of 0.002 ml subcutaneously. The atropine sulphate injection can be diluted 1:10 with sterile water for injection, providing a dose size of 0.02 ml.

ANAESTHESIA

Inhalation anaesthesia

Inhalation anaesthesia is the preferred method and should be used where possible. Methoxyflurane, isoflurane and halothane can all be used in oxygen, or in a 1:1 combination of oxygen and nitrous oxide.

Induction can be carried out in an induction chamber, and once anaesthesia has been induced, the mouse can be maintained on oxygen via a face mask.

Anaesthetic	Induction concentration	Maintenance concentration
Methoxyflurane	3.5–4%	0.5–1%
Halothane	3%	1.5–2%
Isoflurane	3.5–4%	2–2.5%

Ether

Ether should not be used because it is highly irritant to the respiratory passages.

Injection anaesthesia

Injection anaesthesia can also be used. Accurate dosing is essential. The patient must be weighed before the administration of anaesthetic. The size of the patient precludes intravenous administration, and anaesthetics are given by means of intraperitoneal injections using an insulin syringe for greatest accuracy. The response of individual mice to the anaesthetic is variable, so caution must be exercised when calculating dosages.

Ketamine can be given alone or in combination with xylazine or medetomidine. The latter combination has the advantage that anaesthesia can be reversed using atipamezole. The combinations can be given separately, or mixed in the same syringe, and given by intraperitoneal injection.

Ketamine/xylazine

Ketaset (Willows Francis Ltd.)

This contains 100 mg/ml ketamine.

Rompun (Bayer Ltd.)

This contains 20 mg/ml xylazine.

Dose: 150 mg/kg ketamine plus 10 mg/kg xylazine can be given by intraperitoneal injection.

Ketamine/medetomidine

Ketaset (Willows Francis Ltd.)

This contains 100 mg/ml ketamine.

Domitor (Pfizer Ltd.)

This contains 1 mg/ml medetomidine.

Dose: 150 mg/kg ketamine plus 0.5 mg/kg medetomidine can be given by intraperitoneal injection.

Comment: This combination can be reversed with atipamezole (Antisedan, Pfizer Ltd.) at a dose of 1 mg/kg given by either subcutaneous or intraperitoneal injection.

Ketamine

Ketamine can be given alone to provide sedation at a dose of 40 mg/kg by intramuscular injection.

Comment: Even when an injectable anesthetic is used, it is recommended that oxygen should be administered through the face mask during the operative procedure.

ANALGESIA

Buprenorphine

Vetergesic (Animalcare Ltd.)

This contains 0.3 mg/ml buprenorphine.

Dose: 0.2 mg/kg by subcutaneous injection every 8–12 hours. An average 30 g mouse can be given 0.02 ml of Vetergesic.

Paracetamol paediatric syrup

Calpol (Wellcome Ltd.)

The six plus suspension of Calpol contains 50 mg/ml paracetamol.

Dose: 300 mg/kg paracetamol; an average sized mouse would need 9 mg. A 30 g mouse could be given 0.18 ml Calpol orally every 4 hours as required.

POST-OPERATIVE CARE

After anaesthesia a respiratory stimulant can be given. Doxapram (Dopram V, Willows Francis Ltd.) contains 20 mg/ml doxapram and can be given at a dose of 10–15 mg/kg by subcutaneous or intramuscular injection. Oxygen can also be administered via the face mask. Warmth can be provided by an external heat source such as a light bulb.

Fluid replacement

Fluid replacement is important post-surgery, and at any other time when dehydration is a symptom. The fluid of choice is glucose saline (0.9% NaCl, 5% glucose) and this should be warmed to body temperature before being given by subcutaneous injection. The quantity for a mouse is 1–2 ml. No more than 0.5 ml should be given at one site.

INJECTION PROCEDURES

Subcutaneous injections can be made in the scruff of the neck, and up to 2–3 ml fluid can be given by this route.

Intramuscular injections can be given into the quadriceps using a 25 gauge needle. The maximum volume that can be given in this site is 0.05 ml.

Intraperitoneal injections can be made with a 25 gauge needle. The mouse should be held on its back with one hind leg extended. The needle can be introduced along the line of this leg into the centre of the corresponding posterior quadrant of the abdomen; 1–2 ml of fluid can be given by this route.

Intravenous injections are very difficult because of the small size of the patient; the lateral tail vein is used for this procedure.

DRUG TREATMENTS

It is important that the patient's weight is known for dose rate calculations. Because the dose of most treatments is minute, an insulin syringe should be used for greatest accuracy. The mouse has a high metabolic rate, and in some circumstances higher doses may be required together with greater frequency of administration to take account of this.

Antibiotics

When selecting an antibiotic it is better to use one with a broad spectrum of action, and although penicillin may be less toxic for mice than other rodents, an alternative antibiotic is preferred.

When giving antibiotics via the drinking water it may help to sweeten the water to increase its palatability. A little glucose or blackcurrant syrup, e.g. Ribena, can be added.

Tx 1. Ampicillin

Amfipen 15% Injection (Mycofarm)

This contains 150 mg/ml ampicillin.

Dose: 100 mg/kg by subcutaneous injection. For an average mouse this is approximately 0.02 ml. Treatment should be twice daily.

Comment: Although penicillin may be less toxic for mice than other rodents, an alternative antibiotic having a broad spectrum of action is preferred.

Tx 2. Enrofloxacin

Baytril (Bayer plc)

Dose: 10 mg/kg daily.
The 2.5% injection solution can be given subcutaneously at a dose of 0.01 ml/day. The 2.5% oral solution can be diluted 1:1 with blackcurrant syrup and given from a dropper bottle at a dose of 1 drop twice daily.

Drinking water can be medicated with the 2.5% oral solution to produce a concentration of 100 mg/litre by taking 4 ml and making it up to 1 litre with water.

Tx 3. Neomycin

Neobiotic Aquadrops (Upjohn Ltd.)

These contain 50 mg/ml neomycin sulphate.

Dose: The drinking water can be medicated at a rate of 2 g/litre. This concentration can be achieved by diluting 1 ml Aquadrops with 24 ml water.

Tx 4. Potentiated sulphonamides

Borgal 7.5% (Hoechst UK Ltd.)

This injection contains 62.5 mg/ml sulfadoxine and 12.5 mg/ml trimethoprim.

Dose: 1.5 ml/kg by subcutaneous injection. An average 30 g mouse should receive 0.04 ml.

Tribrissen 24% (Mallinckrodt Veterinary Ltd.)

This injectable form contains 40 mg/ml trimethoprim and 200 mg/ml sulphadiazine.

Dose: It can be given orally in the drinking water at a dilution of 1:500, i.e. 1 ml made up to 0.5 litre with drinking water.

Tx 5. Sulphadimidine

Intradine (Norbrook Labs Ltd.)

This contains sulphadimidine 33% w/v.

Dose: The required concentration in the drinking water is 0.2%. This dilution is achieved by taking 6 ml of Intradine and making it up to 1 litre with water.

Tx 6. Oxytetracycline

This antibiotic comes in various presentations, including a powder that can be mixed with water to make an oral solution, and short- and long-acting injectable preparations.

Terramycin LA Injectable (Pfizer Ltd.)

This is a long acting injection containing 200 mg/ml oxytetracycline.

Dose: 60 mg/kg by subcutaneous or intramuscular injection every 3 days. For an average 30 g mouse this approximates to a dose of 0.01 ml.

Engemycin Injection 5% (Mycofarm Ltd.)

This is a short acting injection containing 50 mg/ml oxytetracycline.

Dose: 100 mg/kg by subcutaneous injection daily. A dose for an average 30 g mouse is 0.06 ml.

Terramycin Soluble Powder 5.5% (Pfizer Ltd.)

This contains approximately 200 mg oxytetracycline in one level scoopful (about 4 g) of powder.

Dose: The required concentration is 3 mg/ml. One level scoopful can be dissolved in 66 ml water to achieve this concentration.

Tx 7. Hexachlorophane

Ster-zac Powder (Houghs Healthcare Ltd.)

This contains 0.33% hexachlorophane, 3% zinc oxide and sterilised talc. It is effective in preventing staphylococcal infection.

Ectoparasitic preparations

Tx 8. Amitraz

Aludex (Hoechst UK Ltd.)

This contains 50 g/litre amitraz.

Dose: The recommended concentration is 0.01% (100 ppm) amitraz. This is achieved by diluting 1 ml Aludex in 0.5 litre of water. The solution should be used as a dip, and not rinsed.

Tx 9. Ivermectin

Ivomec Injection for Cattle (Merck, Sharpe & Dolimei)

This is an anti-parasitic injection, effective against both ecto- and endo-parasites containing 1% w/v ivermectin.

Dose: 200 μg/kg. Ivomec can be diluted 1:100, and a dose of 0.06 ml given by subcutaneous injection.

Alternatively Ivomec can be given orally at a dose of 1 drop by mouth (undiluted).

Treatment should be repeated after 10 days.

Tx 10. Fipronil

Frontline (Rhône Mérieux)

This spray contains 0.25% w/v fipronil.

Dose: A concentration of 7.5 mg/kg can be used; it may be necessary to dilute with isopropyl alcohol to achieve this dose rate. The treatment may be repeated monthly.

Tx 11. Pyrethrin

Anti-mite Spray for Birds (Johnson)

This contains 0.8% w/v pyrethrin and piperonyl.

Dose: A light spray may be given and repeated weekly if necessary.

Endoparasitic preparations

Tx 12. Niclosamide

This is an anti-parasitic drug effective against cestodes.

Troscan 100 (Bayer plc.)

These tablets contains 100 mg niclosamide, and one thirtieth of a tablet can be given to an adult mouse, and the dose repeated after 7 days. This approximates to a dose of 100 mg/kg.

Tx 13. Piperazine

This is an anti-parasitic drug effective against roundworms.

Antepar Elixir (Wellcome)

Antepar contains 150 mg/ml piperazine and this will control nematodes (pinworms).

Dose: The required concentration of 3 mg/ml piperazine in the drinking water can be achieved by diluting the exlixir 1:50 with water, and replacing the drinking water with this solution.

Corticosteroids

Tx 14. Betamethasone

Betsolan Injection (Mallinckrodt Veterinary Ltd.)

This contains 2 mg/ml betamethasone.

Dose: 0.1 mg/kg by subcutaneous injection. For an average mouse this approximates to 0.002 ml.

Tx 15. Dexamethasone

Dexadreson (Intervet UK Ltd.)

This contains a rapid action formulation of dexamethasone at a concentration of 2 mg/ml.

Dose: 0.5 mg/kg dexamethasone can be given by subcutaneous injection.

Antigungal agents

Tx 16. Griseofulvin

Grisovin (Mallinckrodt Veterinary Ltd.)

This is an antifungal treatment for the treatment of ringworm. Each Grisovin tablet contains 125 mg of griseofulvin.

Dose: Treatment should be continued for at least a month, at a dose of 25 mg/kg orally. Two tablets could be ground to a powder and evenly mixed with a month's food ration to provide the required dose.

Tx 17. Enilconazole

Imaverol (Jansen)

This contains 100 mg/ml enilconazole.

Dose: This can be diluted 1:50 to provide a 0.2% w/v solution which can be used as a weekly dip.

Miscellaneous treatments

Tx 18. Kaolin/pectin

Kaogel (Parke Davis & Co. Ltd.)

Kaogel contains 20% w/v light kaolin and 0.43% w/v pectin.

Dose: One drop orally three times daily, as an adjunct to other diarrhoea therapy.

Comment: Many paediatric diarrhoea preparations are similar, and make suitable alternatives.

Tx 19. Metronidazole

Metronidazole is an antibiotic with anti-protozoal activity.

Torgyl solution (Rhône Mérieux Ltd.)

This contains 5 mg/ml metronidazole and can be diluted 1:1 with drinking water to provide a concentration of 2.5 mg/ml.

Flagyl-s Solution (May and Baker)

This contains 40 mg/ml metronidazole and can be diluted 1:16 with drinking water to produce a concentration of 2.5 mg/ml.

Tx 20. Aspirin

Dose: 120 mg/kg; for a 30 g mouse this is 3.6 mg. Soluble aspirin could be given in the drinking water at a concentration of 1 mg/ml.

Tx 21. Paracetamol

Calpol (Wellcome)

This contains 50 mg/ml paracetamol.

Dose: 300 mg/kg; an average sized mouse (30 g) would need 9 mg, and could be given 0.18 ml Calpol orally every 4 hours as required.

Tx 22. Multivitamin preparation

Abidec Drops (Parke Davis)

These contain vitamins A, B_1 (thiamine), B_2, B_6, niacin, C and D. They can be given by mouth or added to the drinking water.

Dose: One drop daily is sufficient for an average mouse.

Topical preparations

Tx 23. Sudocrem (Tosara Products Ltd.)

This is a zinc oxide cream in a liquid paraffin base.

Tx 24. Dermisol (Pfizer Ltd.)

This ointment contains propylene glycol, malic acid, benzoic acid and salicylic acid. It promotes healing by removing dead and necrotic tissue from affected areas and also has antibacterial properties. It can be applied two or three times daily.

Eye preparations

Tx 25. Chlortetracycline

Aureomycin Ophthalmic Ointment (Cyanamid Ltd.)

This contains 1% w/v chlortetracycline.

RATS

There are two species of rat most commonly encountered, *Rattus norvegicus* the brown rat, and *Rattus rattus* the black rat. It is *Rattus norvegicus* which has become adapted to the fancy rat that is kept today. Rats first appeared in the western world in the eighteenth century from China, and were kept as both fancy and laboratory animals. Although rat shows were held at the beginning of the twentieth century, the Fancy Rat Society was only formed in 1976.

The standard colour is agouti, with a white or cream underbelly. A wide variety of solid and patterned coat colours have now been developed, as has the rex coat type.

16 HUSBANDRY AND NUTRITION

Environment

Small numbers of rats may be kept indoors, whilst larger numbers can be accommodated in an outhouse. Wherever they are kept the ventilation should be good, and the accommodation should be free from damp and draughts. The ideal external temperature is between 15 and 27°C (59–80°F), with a relative humidity of 40–70%. The rats should be kept out of direct sunlight which may cause heatstroke in the warmer months. At temperatures above 30°C (86°F) heatstroke is likely, especially if the rats are overstocked. Bright lights have also been shown to damage the retinas, particularly of albino rats.

Rats should not be kept in garages with a car because the exhaust fumes will be toxic. Whatever the environment it must be free from predators, and protected against the entry of wild rats and mice. A dichlorvos strip, e.g. Vapona, can be hung close to the cages, and this will reduce the number of flies in the surrounding environment; it will also reduce the number of any external parasites.

Housing

A single pet rat is likely to be kept indoors, and its accommodation should be clean, secure and odour-free. Wire cages or glass or plastic aquariums are most commonly used. However, breeders with larger numbers of rats may keep them in a variety of cages, including hutches or plastic crates. The minimum size is 45 cm × 30 cm × 25 cm (l × w × h). The rat is a keen gnawer, and any cage should be secure.

Wire cages offer good ventilation, but care must be taken to ensure the rat does not get its legs trapped in the wire, and subsequently damaged. If the cage is made of galvanised steel, and the rat chews the bars, it may get zinc poisoning from the bars.

Aquariums must be regularly cleaned, as they offer less ventilation, and any build up of ammonia from the urine will predispose to respiratory disease.

Wooden hutches should be strong and, because they are likely to be gnawed, made only of untreated woods.

The floorspace can be increased by introducing extra levels within the cage, linked by ladders or tubing.

The accommodation must be placed out of direct sunlight; aquariums, in particular, will rapidly become hot in the summer.

Bedding

The most common floor litter is wood shavings. These should be made from pine or softwoods because those made from cedar or hard woods are likely to be toxic. The cage floor should be covered to a depth of 1 cm. Bedding is also required, for which shredded paper can be used, although shredded newspaper is not recommended because the inks from the print may be toxic, and stain the coat. Good quality dry straw and hay can also be used for bedding.

Although the floor litter and bedding should be adsorbent, they should not be so drying as to reduce the relative humidity below 40% because certain conditions, such as ringtail and respiratory disease, are more prevalent at low humidities. Fine sawdust may predispose to allergies and respiratory disease.

Stocking

Pet rats can live singly or in pairs. Adult males may fight, but single sex siblings may live together in harmony, particularly if kept together from weaning. The larger the cage size the better, as overcrowding is a stress which predisposes to disease.

Nutrition

General principles

Rats are omnivores, and can be fed both meat and plants. They will eat practically anything, but the best growth rates and body weight are achieved if the basic diet is a high protein (around 24%) mix. The diet of an adult rat should contain only 14% protein for maintenance; this may need to be raised to 24% for optimum breeding efficiency. Rats can be fed proprietary pellets, or mixes. A dry complete dog or cat food with similar protein level is also suitable. Hamster mixes are less suitable because they contain sunflower seeds and peanuts which are high in protein and oil, and cause skin allergies and spots. Specific rat mixes contain no seeds or nuts, to avoid skin problems.

The diet can be supplemented with fresh fruit and vegetables, cooked eggs, and dog biscuits. Cooked chicken and fish can also be given as sources of easily digestible protein, and carbohydrates can be supplied in the form of bread and oats.

Because rats will eat almost anything, care must be taken not to offer treats or biscuits too often as this will rapidly lead to obesity. Chocolate in large quantities is toxic to rats. Sugary foods may be good for tempting the appetite of a sick rat, but an excess will cause diarrhoea.

Vitamin supplementation of healthy rats is unnecessary; rats are able to synthesise their own vitamin C, and satisfy their vitamin B requirements by coprophagy.

Food should be supplied in a solid bowl that cannot be tipped, spilled or chewed. Water should be permanently available from a sipper bottle. The average water intake is 10 ml/100 g body weight daily.

Protein

An excess of protein can cause skin allergies and spots. A diet deficient in protein will cause hair loss, porphyrin staining around the eyes, and pre-dispose towards infections. Pregnant and lactating females, and youngsters under the age of 4 months have the highest protein requirements (at least 24%). The protein requirement of an adult rat for maintenance is 14% and this can be provided by a rat or rabbit mix, or complete dry food for older dogs.

Milk can be given from weaning at 4–6 weeks until 8 weeks, either as cow's milk, or a powdered form for puppies (e.g. Lactol).

Obesity

Care must be taken when feeding biscuits and treats that the rats do not become obese. Obesity will lead to a shorter life span, poorer breeding capacity and sore hocks. Tumour development is also more common in obese animals.

Obesity can be corrected by feeding a ration restricted in calories, and introducing more fruit and vegetables. Exercise should also be encouraged. Calorie restriction has also been shown to increase life span and reduce the incidence of neoplasia.

17 SYSTEMS AND DISEASES

THE SKIN

Abscesses

These generally occur as a result of fighting, but may also occur spontaneously in older or debilitated rats.

Treatment: The abscess should be lanced and drained, under anaesthesia if necessary. Antibiotics (Tx 1–6) should be given orally for extensive abscesses, or used topically for minor wounds. Dermisol cream (Tx 17) can also be used topically.

Ectoparasites

Lice

Rats can be infected by the sucking louse *Polyplax spinulosa*. Clinical signs include pruritus and alopecia, particularly around the head and neck. General failure to thrive and agitation is seen with heavy infestations.

Treatment: Pyrethrin, either as a powder or spray (Tx 23) can be applied weekly as necessary. Ivermectin (Tx 11) can also be given orally.

The toenails should be trimmed to prevent self-excoriation.

Dichlorvos strips, e.g. Vapona, can be hung close to the cage and are effective in reducing ectoparasite numbers.

The cage should be thoroughly cleaned, and can also be sprayed with a pyrethrin spray (Tx 23).

Fleas

Rats can be infested with fleas from wild rodents, or in-contact cats and dogs. Treatment with a pyrethrin product is effective. Dichlorvos strips, e.g. Vapona, can be hung near the cage to repel fleas.

Mange

Sarcoptic mange causes intense pruritus and alopecia, especially over the dorsum. Crusty sores occur behind the ears and on the neck. Clinical signs are worst if the immune system is compromised, as in old, debilitated or undernourished individuals. Diagnosis is by the examination of skin scrapings.

Treatment: Ivermectin (Tx 11) can be given either orally or by injection, and the treatment repeated every 10–14 days. Affected rats can also be dipped in a 0.01% solution of amitraz (Tx 12. Aludex). Dipping should be repeated weekly for at least 6 weeks.

Ringworm

This is usually caused by *Microsporum* spp. which fluoresce under a Wood's lamp.

Clinical signs: Scaly areas of alopecia, which may become inflamed, are seen Ringworm is occasionally pruritic; it can be diagnosed by microscopy and culture, or by its fluorescence with a Woods lamp. Some rats may be long-term carriers without showing clinical signs, and can only be identified by culture of hair brushings.

Treatment: Griseofulvin (Tx 9) should be given at a dose of 25 mg/kg daily for 4–6 weeks. Affected animals can also be washed with chlorhexidine 1%, and then dipped in 0.2% enilconazole. Imaverol (Tx 10) contains 100 mg/ml enilconazole and can be diluted 1:50 to provide the 0.2% solution. Treatment can be repeated weekly.

Alopecia

Barbering of cage mates is relatively uncommon. The dominant rat can be detected as it will be the only one unaffected; it should be removed.

Diets that are too high in protein and oil will cause alopecia and a skin rash. Dietary allergies will also cause similar symptoms. The diet of an adult rat should contain 14% protein, and no nuts or sunflower seeds. If an allergy is suspected any coloured pieces in the mix should be excluded. More fruit and vegetables should be slowly introduced to the daily ration.

Allergic dermatitis may also occur as a response to bedding, cigarette smoke, and household sprays. Allergic rhinitis may also occur. The bedding should be changed from sawdust or shavings to shredded white paper.

Non-specific pruritus can be treated with doses of systemic corticosteroids (Tx 8).

Ringtail

This occurs if the relative humidity drops below 40%. Other predisposing factors are excessive ventilation, and over-adsorbent bedding. The tail develops annular constrictions, which may lead to necrosis and sloughing. Young rats (7–15 days old) are most commonly affected. The relative humidity should be raised to a minimum of 50%, and ideally 70%.

Ringtail is most commonly seen in the winter when the external environment is heated and the humidity may drop. It may in part be prevented by housing the young litters in solid plastic-bottomed cages with adequate nesting and bedding material.

Skin tumours

These are very common in older rats, and obese animals are most prone to their development. Most common are fibroadenomas of the mammary glands, and these can grow rapidly to a size which hinders locomotion. Surgical removal is possible in the early stages, but recurrence is common. These tumours are usually benign; it is their size and weight which cause clinical problems.

Much less common are squamous cell carcinomas around the head. Squamous cell carcinomas can also develop in the Zymbal's gland of the external ear.

Seborrhoea

As the rat ages the grease glands may become more active, and a greasy coat is more common in older animals. No treatment is necessary, although shampooing with an antidandruff preparation will relieve the symptoms.

Rough coat

Older rats kept alone, or malnourished rats may have a rough coat. A leaking water bottle, soiled bedding or diarrhoea may all also lead to the development of a rough, stary coat.

THE REPRODUCTIVE SYSTEM

- Litter size: average 10
- Birth weight: 6 g
- Weaning: 4 weeks
- Puberty: 8–10 weeks
- Oestrus cycle: 4–5 days
- Duration of oestrus: 12–24 hours
- Post-partum oestrus: is fertile 24 hours after parturition
- Gestation: 20–22 days

Sexing

Sexing is possible from a young age. In males the anogenital distance is twice as long as that of the female (Figure 17.1). In males the testes descend early, and if the male is held with his head up the testes are visible in the scrotal sac. The female nipples may be evident from 10–15 days of age.

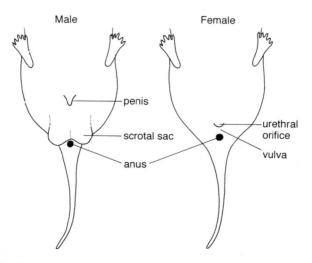

Figure 17.1   External genitalia.

Stocking

Rats can be kept as a breeding pair, or one male rat can be kept with a group of between two and six females in a polygamous system. If rats are kept as a group they must be allowed plenty of space, because over-crowding may lead to stress, apparent infertility or cannibalism of litters.

If a male and female are to be paired only for mating the female must be introduced to the male's cage and not vice versa. Alternatively the pair can be introduced on neutral territory.

Puberty and breeding

Rats reach puberty between 2 and 3 months of age, when their body weight is 250–300 g. They are best mated for the first time at 4–$4\frac{1}{2}$ months of age. The females have oestrus cycles all year round, each cycle lasting 4–5 days, during which time they are receptive to the male for approximately 14 hours. If several females are housed together they may all exhibit oestrus simultaneously (the Whitten effect). Signs of oestrus are lordosis, and a willingness to be mounted by the male; the vulva is open and a purple colour. After mating a waxy plug (the copulatory plug) fills the vagina. This plug, which contains secretions from the male accessory sex glands, prevents leakage of semen from the vagina; it drops out after 24 hours, and if found is a sign that mating has taken place.

Gestation

Gestation lasts 20–22 days. Pregnancy may be determined by gentle abdominal palpation from day 15, or by weighing to record a weight gain. Mammary development becomes more pronounced in the last third of gestation. The female should be separated by the sixteenth day of gestation, because if the male is present at the birth he may cannibalise or desert the young, or agalactia may result. The female also exhibits a fertile post-partum oestrus 24 hours after parturition, but a breed-back at this stage will rapidly drain the female's reserves.

The female will begin nest building 2–3 days before the birth.

If the gestation is the result of a post-partum mating, and the pregnant female is lactating, the gestation period may be extended by 2–3 days.

Delayed implantation can occur for up to 7–10 days, giving an apparent gestation period of 28–30 days. As long as the female is well and there is no abnormal vaginal discharge a longer gestation can be considered to be the result of delayed implantation, rather than an overdue pregnancy.

Complications during pregnancy

Abortion and miscarriage

This may occur if the female is kept in poor environmental conditions, is poorly nourished, or has an underlying disease. Abortion and miscarriage may go unnoticed as the female will eat any dead fetuses or fetal material. However, she may develop a vaginal discharge, which if unpleasant is a symptom of uterine infection. If endometritis or pyometritis is suspected antibiotics should be given systemically.

Pseudopregnancy

This is rare, but if it occurs it lasts 13 days, after which time the female returns to oestrus.

Parturition

Parturition generally occurs at night. The first stage of labour begins with the loss of a clear vaginal discharge which the female will lick. The second stage, the delivery of the young, generally takes $1\frac{1}{2}$ hours. The young are born naked, with their eyes and ears closed. The female should not be disturbed for the first 2–3 days post-partum as she may abandon or cannibalise the young.

Problems during or after parturition

Perineal tears

A slight vaginal discharge post-partum is normal, but if there is heavy bleeding, or if the doe repeatedly licks her vulva, she should be carefully examined. Does may aquire perineal tears during parturition which may require the administration of antibiotic (Tx 1), either orally or topically.

Mastitis

This is not common, and must be differentiated from mammary neoplasia.

The affected gland will be swollen, warm, and may ulcerate. The causal agent may be *Staphylococcus* or *Pasteurella pneumotropica*.

Treatment: The gland can be bathed with warm poultices, and antibiotics (Tx 1–6) given orally or systemically. If there are areas of ulceration these should be kept clean and a topical preparation (Tx 17. Dermisol) applied.

Weaning

The young develop rapidly, and by 10 days of age have their eyes and ears open, and a covering of hair. Weaning takes place at 3–4 weeks when the average weight of the young is 45 g.

The young should be raised on a food with 24% protein content, and some cow's milk or puppy replacement milk can be given for the first 2–3 weeks.

The female rat returns to oestrus cycling 2–4 days after weaning.

Problems with the male

Preputial gland abscess

These occur in the male, and are seen as bilateral swellings around the penis. The causal agents are usually *Staphylococcus aureus* or *Pasteurella pneumotropica*. A unilateral swelling may indicate a much rarer neoplasm.

Treatment: The abscesses should be lanced and drained under anaesthesia. Antibiotics (Tx 1–6) can be given systemically or orally. A tumour of the preputial gland should be removed surgically.

Testicular tumours

Male rats may develop interstitial cell tumours of the testes. On examination the testicles will be of uneven size, the larger often hard and swollen. These tumours do not metastasize and castration is curative.

Surgical procedures

Castration

Rats have open inguinal canals, and the testes can move between the scrotum and the abdomen. If the testes are not visible, gentle pressure on the abdomen should push them into the scrotum. The testes can be removed via a pre-scrotal incision, the vas deferens and spermatic cord blood vessels ligated, and the inguinal canal closed. The lining of the scrotum and the skin should be closed in two separate layers.

Ovariohysterectomy

This should be performed through a mid-line incision. The ovarian vessels must be ligated, and the uterine vessels ligated with the cervix. The abdominal and skin incisions should be closed routinely.

Fostering

Orphans can be fostered successfully onto a mother with a litter of the same age. The orphans should be rubbed in the bedding of the foster family so that they smell the same and are less likely to be rejected. Hand rearing is also possible, but difficult; aspiration pneumonia or chilling are very common.

Infertility

- Rats are most fertile between 3 and 10 months of age, after which time they may take longer to conceive, and have smaller litters. Female rats may stop having oestrus cycles at around 15 months of age. Male rats are capable of breeding for their whole life. Occasionally, a male may have one or both testicles which remain in the abdomen undescended, and these males may have reduced fertility or be infertile. The condition is thought to be hereditary and they should not be used to breed.
- Overcrowding or poor nutrition, concurrent disease or ectoparasitism may lead to a cessation of breeding until conditions are improved.
- Other environmental factors, such as high temperature or humidity, or constant light may also cause infertility. A 12 hour light/12 hour darkness regime is recommended for maximum breeding success.

- Vitamin E deficiency. Wheatgerm is a good source of this vitamin, and this can be regularly sprinkled on the food.
- Low protein diets. Although the protein requirement for maintenance of the adult rat is 14% this may need to be raised to 24% for optimum breeding efficiency.

THE URINARY SYSTEM

Chronic renal failure

This is very common in older rats, the onset of the condition occurring as early as 12–14 months of age. It occurs most commonly in rats fed refined, high protein diets.

Clinical signs: These include polydipsia, polyuria, proteinuria and, as the condition progresses, hydrothorax and ascites.

Treatment: By the time clinical signs are evident the kidney damage is present, and treatment is of little value. It may help to feed a lower protein ration, and mix in boiled rice to the diet to slow the progress of renal failure.

Cystitis

This is an uncommon finding.

Clinical signs: These are haematuria and discomfort on urination. Haematuria is also a symptom of urinary calculi or bladder neoplasia. Calculi or neoplasia may be diagnosed by palpation and radiography.

Treatment: Cystitis can be successfully treated with antibiotics (Tx 1–6) given either systemically or orally.

Parasitic infection of the bladder

The nematode *Trichosomoides crassicauda* has the rat as its only host. The female nematode lives in the bladder and can grow to a length of 9–10 mm. The male nematode lives permanently in the reproductive tract of the female rat. The female nematode attaches herself to the bladder lining and passes eggs out in the urine.

Clinical signs: Mild infections cause no problems, but the bladder irritation that can be caused may lead to cystitis, calculi or neoplasia. Severe calculi may lead to dysuria and loss of condition.

Diagnosis: The eggs can be identified in the urine, and associated calculi may be palpable.

Treatment: Ivermectin (Tx 11) can be given orally, and the dose repeated after 10–14 days.

Leptospirosis

This is uncommon in pet rats unless they have been exposed to wild rodent carriers. Rats can harbour patent leptospire infections without showing any clinical signs. The disease is a zoonosis, and infection can be spread from secretions of nose, mouth and urine of carriers to humans through skin abrasions.

Diagnosis: This is via urine culture or serology.

Clinical signs (human infection): These include non-specific malaise, fever, headaches and myalgia, influenza-like symptoms. There may be an associated skin rash and conjunctivitis.

Comment: Because of the severe zoonotic risk any affected animals and also their cages and bedding should be destroyed (see Zoonotic Aspects). It is important that pet rats should never come into contact with wild rodents.

THE DIGESTIVE SYSTEM

THE TEETH

Malocclusion

Uneven wear and overgrowth of the incisors can occur following trauma, developmental problems or occasionally may be hereditary. If there is damage to a tooth root so that it fails to grow, the corresponding incisor on the opposite jaw will not be worn down, and will overgrow. Similarly if a tooth is broken, tooth overgrowth can occur. If overgrowth is unchecked the lower incisors can grow into the palate. Rat incisors are capable of growing 10–12 cm a year and rely on the process of gnawing to keep them worn down.

Treatment: The incisors may need to be regularly trimmed to promote even wear, and hard food such as dog biscuits or dry macaroni can be given to encourage gnawing.

Dental caries

Rats will eat almost anything and will pick out sweet treats, cakes and biscuits before eating their staple mix. Although sweets may be given to aid training, they should be limited because their consumption leads to dental caries.

Treatment: It is possible to extract incisors if a root abscess develops, but the remaining incisors will need regular trimming because, with one or more teeth missing, the wear will be uneven.

THE OESOPHAGUS

Megaoesophagus

This has been recorded in hooded rats.

Clinical signs: These include dyspnoea associated with inhalation pneumonia, and the presence of food around the mouth. The diagnosis can be confirmed by a barium X-ray which would highlight the dilated oesophagus. The prognosis is poor.

THE STOMACH AND INTESTINES

Endoparasites

Infection with intestinal parasites is common, but clinical disease associated with endoparasites is rare, and seen only in young or immunosuppressed animals with very heavy burdens. The commonest endoparasites are *Hymenolepis nana*, *Hymenolepis diminuta* (rat tapeworm) and the pinworm *Syphacia muris*.

Tapeworm

Clinical signs: Large burdens in the young may cause weight loss, intestinal obstruction and death. The eggs are present on faecal examination.

Treatment: Niclosamide (Tx 15) is effective.

Hymenolepis diminuta has an indirect life cycle using a flea or beetle. It can easily be eradicated by vector control, together with regular cleaning of the cage and changing of the bedding to remove any eggs that are shed.

Hymenolepis nana also uses beetles as hosts, but also has a life cycle which involves the tapeworm egg developing in the original host, and undergoing tissue migration, making eradication harder.

Pinworm

Clinical signs: Diarrhoea, rectal prolapse, and poor condition may be seen in young animals with high worm burdens. The banana-shaped eggs can be collected from the anal area with sticky tape and identified by microscopy.

Treatment: Ivermectin (Tx 11) or piperazine (Tx 16) are effective. The pinworm has a direct life cycle; the female migrates from the bowel and lays eggs on the skin. The eggs are ingested by the host, and mature to adults in the bowel.

Protozoa

Trichomonas and Giardia

Protozoa may be identified on examination of faecal samples, but are generally considered non-pathogenic. Very large burdens may cause enteritis. The commonest protozoa are *Trichomonas muris*, and *Giardia muris*.

Treatment: Metronidazole (Tx 14) is effective and can be put in the drinking water at a concentration of 2.5 mg/ml.

Coccidia

Coccidia spp. are also found and considered non-pathogenic. Large numbers of *Eimeria* may cause disease if husbandry methods are poor.

Treatment: Coccidia can be treated with sulphadimidine (Tx 5) for a week.

Diarrhoea

Diarrhoea may be dietary, or associated with endoparasites or bacterial infection (*Salmonella*, Tyzzer's disease).

Dietary

Dietary upset from the feeding of too many treats or green food results in loose motions, although the affected rat is usually bright and still eating.

Treatment: A kaolin/pectin (Tx 13) preparation can be given orally. Green food should be stopped, and burnt toast or arrowroot biscuits can be offered.

Salmonellosis

Clinical signs: These include diarrhoea, dry coat, unthriftiness and sudden death. The organism *Salmonella enteritidis* is identified on faecal culture.

Salmonellosis is a zoonosis, and if the disease is confirmed affected animals should be culled. The cage and utensils should be disinfected; floor litter and bedding should be destroyed (see Zoonotic Aspects). It is very important to prevent exposure of pet rats to wild rodents because they are the carriers of the infection.

Tyzzer's disease

This is caused by the bacterium *Clostridium piliforme*. Bacterial spores are shed in the faeces; these spores are resistant to most disinfectants, and only destroyed by high temperatures and dilute bleach. Tyzzer's disease may be triggered by poor environments, stress and overcrowding.

Clinical signs: Ruffled dry coat, hunched posture, diarrhoea and bloated abdomen. On necropsy pale grey foci are evident on the liver.

Treatment: Supportive therapy, warmth, fluids and the administration of a kaolin/pectin mixture (Tx 13) are required.

Oxytetracycline (Tx 6) in the drinking water can help control and prevent the spread of infection.

THE RESPIRATORY SYSTEM

Respiratory disease is one of the commonest problems for rats, it may be insidious on onset, or it may be triggered by stress. The rat has Harderian glands in the eyes which produce porphyrin secretions in response to stress ('red tears'). Respiratory disease may affect the upper respiratory tract the (eyes, ears and nose), or the lower respiratory tract (the lungs).

Rats are exposed to numerous bacteria and viruses responsible for respiratory infection, and many rats have subclinical infections and lung lesions in the absence of any clinical signs. However, stress in the form of overcrowding, poor nutrition or a build up of ammonia from urine may trigger disease. The administration of an anaesthetic is a significant trigger for lower respiratory infection if lung lesions are already present.

Any decision on treatment must take into consideration the numbers of animals involved and the number of in-contact animals at risk. Pet animals can be usually treated successfully, although there is likely to be some residual lung damage. If large numbers of in-contact rats are at risk it may be best to cull affected rats.

The commonest agents involved in respiratory disease are *Pasteurella pneumotropica*, *Bordetella bronchiseptica* and *Mycoplasma pulmonis*.

Upper respiratory tract disease

Clinical signs: There is red porphyrin staining (not blood) of the eyes and nose, face rubbing, and sneezing. Occasionally a head tilt to one side is evident.

Lower respiratory tract disease

Clinical signs: Dyspnoea and wheezing occur; also anorexia, weight loss and lethargy are seen. The rat adopts a hunched posture.

Treatment: The rat should be isolated in warm and clean surroundings. Antibiotics (Tx 1–6) should be given orally or systemically. Where there is accompanying conjunctivitis the eyes should be bathed, and an eye preparation (Tx 18, 21, 22) used. If the rat is rubbing its face the best bedding to use is shredded white paper, because sawdust will further irritate the eyes, and may lead to corneal ulceration and oedema.

Mentholated ointment (e.g. Vick) can be rubbed on the side of the hospital cage.

Specific agents of respiratory disease

Mycoplasma

The causal agent is *Mycoplasma pulmonis*. Infection may be sub-clinical, or there may be upper and lower respiratory symptoms, and torticollis if there is inner ear infection. Lung abscesses are often present, and occasionally there may be associated endometritis.

The disease is triggered by high ammonia levels from wet litter, and by concurrent viral infection with the Sendai or sialodacryoadenitis virus.

Treatment: Clinical signs may be suppressed with the antibiotics tylosin (Tx 7) or oxytetracycline (Tx 6), but the carrier state cannot be eliminated. Improvement of cage hygiene will prevent clinical signs developing.

Streptococcal pneumonia

This is caused by the bacterium *Streptococcus pneumoniae*. In small numbers this bacterium forms part of the normal flora of the respiratory tract, but an overwhelming number can cause serious clinical signs.

Clinical signs: A suppurative nasal discharge and fibrinous pneumonia are seen. There may be middle and inner ear infection, with accompanying signs of torticollis and circling. Some animals may develop septicaemia and die.

Treatment: Antibiotics (Tx 1–6) may be administered orally or systemically.

Pseudotuberculosis

The causal agent is *Corynebacterium kutscheri*. Infections are usually subclinical, but some rats may develop lower respiratory tract symptoms associated with abscesses in the lung parenchyma. Clinically unaffected rats may be carriers, and shed the organism.

Treatment: Antibiotics, particularly oxytetracycline (Tx 6) or chloramphenicol (Tx 2) can be used to reduce clinical signs, but it is impossible to eliminate the carrier state.

Coronavirus

Rats can be infected by a coronavirus, sialodacryadenitis virus. Clinical signs depend upon the age and the immunocompetence of the individual. In colonies where sialodacryadenitis virus is endemic young rats will be protected with maternal antibodies, and will only show a mild and transient conjunctivitis when older. In rats that have not been previously exposed to the virus clinical signs are more severe.

Clinical signs: There is inflammation of the salivary glands, lymph nodes and lacrimal glands. There is an increase in red (porphyrin) tear staining of the face. Affected animals recover 1–2 weeks after infection, and mortality is generally low in adults, but higher in youngsters.

Treatment: Supportive therapy is needed whilst recovery takes place. Recovered females will then confer immunity to any further youngsters born.

Pasteurella

Pasteurella pneumotropica is an opportunist bacterium which may be carried in small numbers in healthy rats with no clinical signs. However, if large numbers of bacteria are present with another co-existing respiratory agent, clinical disease may occur.

Clinical signs: Dyspnoea and weight loss are seen, with multiple abscesses in various sites (the lungs, Harderian glands, skin, reproductive tract). The middle ear, eyes (conjunctivitis) and lymph nodes may also be affected.

Treatment: Oral antibiotics may relieve the clinical signs, but will not prevent the carrier state. Chloramphenicol (Tx 2) can be used in the drinking water.

THE EYE

'Red tears'

The eye has a Harderian gland which secretes porphryins ('red tears') in response to stresses such as overcrowding, poor nutrition and concurrent infection, especially a respiratory infection. These tears are often mistaken for blood; they can be examined under an ultraviolet light, and will fluoresce.

If the tears are from one eye only it may indicate a blocked tear duct on that side, or atrophy of the gland on the opposite side.

Treatment: The eye must be bathed and an ophthalmic preparation can be applied. A preparation containing chloramphenicol (Tx 18. Chloromycetin Ophthalmic Ointment) or tetracycline (Tx 20. Aureomycin Ophthalmic Ointment) is suitable. Concurrent respiratory disease must be treated and all stress removed. Any sand or sawdust in the cage must be removed because it could cause further corneal abrasions when the rat burrows.

Conjunctivitis

Inflammation and irritation of the conjunctiva can occur as symptoms of respiratory disease, or as a condition on their own. Conjunctivitis may occur as a result of an allergy to bedding, aerosol sprays or cigarette smoke. A build up of ammonia from damp bedding will also cause severe irritation. The condition may be recurrent.

Clinical signs: Inflammation of the conjunctiva, ocular discharge, face rubbing and hair loss around the eyes may be evident. There is an increase in 'red tears' around the eyes and nose.

Treatment: Ophthalmic ointments or drops (Tx 18, 21, 22) may be used. An antibiotic/steroid preparation may be applied (Tx 19. Chloromycetin Hydrocortisone Ophthalmic Ointment) as long as there is no corneal damage.

Corneal ulceration

Severe irritation of the eye, or coronavirus infection may lead to corneal ulceration, opacity, and occasionally rupture of the globe.

Corneal ulceration should be treated with antibiotic ointment (Tx 18. Chloromycetin Ophthalmic Ointment); more severe eye trauma may naturally enucleate or require surgical enucleation.

Retinal degeneration

Bright lights in the environment have been shown to damage the retinas, particularly of albino rats, and subsequent retinal degeneration will lead to blindness. A rat kept in a familiar environment will be able to cope with loss of vision with few problems.

THE EAR

Middle ear infection

This is a sequel to certain respiratory infections. The rat exhibits torticollis, and may circle to one side. There may be a loss of balance. Treatment with antibiotics (Tx 1–6) may reduce the clinical signs and halt the infection; however, there is often a persistence of the head tilt. The rat may learn to compensate for this and cope adequately. At necropsy the middle ear will be found to be full of debris.

Incoordination may also be seen in older rats associated with a tumour of the pituitary gland. These tumours are common in older rats, and may be asymptomatic until the growth is of a size to act as a space-occupying lesion in the brain. Some rats may also show weight loss.

Zymbal's gland

This gland is found below the ear. It may become neoplastic in the older rat.

THE MUSCULOSKELETAL SYSTEM

Degenerative myelopathy

Rats around the age of 2 years may develop spinal nerve root degeneration and associated muscle degeneration, leading to clinical signs of posterior paresis, paralysis and incoordination. As the rat drags itself on its hind legs it may develop calluses and sores on its legs. The rat is likely to develop urine scalding.

The rat can be kept comfortable on clean soft bedding, but euthanasia should be considered if sores develop, or if the rat is unable to readily reach its food or water.

Fractures

Long bone fractures may result from trauma such as a fall, and can be diagnosed by radiography. It is possible to support-dress closed fractures; however, the rat may attempt to gnaw the dressing and further traumatise the leg. If the fracture is reasonably stable it can be left without support and a callus will form in 7–10 days. The rat must be kept confined in a small cage so it is unable to climb or jump.

Spinal trauma may present with symptoms similar to those of degenerative myelopathy, and must be differentiated from it by radiography.

Pododermatitis

Foot lesions may be seen in rats housed on rough or wire floors, or when there is poor hygiene and soiled bedding.

Treatment: The lesions should be bathed and an antibiotic (Tx 1–6) given, or antiseptic cream (Tx 17. Dermisol) applied. The rat should be moved to a cage with a solid bottom and plenty of clean and soft bedding.

Arthritis

Stiffness of the joints may occur in rats over 2 years of age. Affected rats should be kept comfortable on soft bedding. A drop of cod-liver oil can be added to the food on a daily basis to help alleviate the symptoms.

18 ANAESTHESIA AND DRUG TREATMENTS

HANDLING

Rats can be picked up by placing a hand around their shoulders, and be held firmly enough to steady the patient, but not so tightly that breathing is compromised. Rats resent being scruffed, and may bite in fear. Once lifted out of their cage they can be steadied with the other hand by holding the base of the tail.

PRE-ANAESTHETIC PREPARATION

In common with other rodents rats are unable to vomit, and do not require starving before the administration of an anaesthetic.

Hypothermia during anaesthesia may develop and precautions are necessary too help prevent the loss of body heat by the patient. The rat can be wrapped in silver foil or bubble-wrap for the duration of the anaesthetic and recovery period, or placed on a heat reflective surface, e.g. on a Flectabed.

When the operation site is prepared the rat should not be overwetted because this will increase heat loss by evaporation. All cleaning solutions should be at body temperature.

ANAESTHESIA

Inhalation anaesthesia

Gaseous anesthesia is the preferred method and should be used where possible. Methoxyflurane, isoflurane and halothane can all be used in oxygen, or in a 1:1 combination of oxygen and nitrous oxide.

Induction can be made in an induction chamber, and once anaesthesia is induced, the rat can be maintained on a face mask.

Anaesthetic	Induction concentration	Maintenance concentration
Methoxyflurane	3.5%	0.5–1%
Halothane	3%	1.5–2%
Isoflurane	3.5–4%	2–2.5%

Ether

Ether should not be used as it is highly irritant to the respiratory passages.

Injection anaesthesia

Injectable anaesthetics can also be used. Accurate dosing is essential. The patient must be weighed before the administration of anaesthetic. The size of the patient precludes intravenous administration, and anaesthetics are given by means of intraperitoneal injections using an insulin syringe for greatest accuracy. The response of individual rats to the anaesthetic is variable, so caution must be exercised when calculating dosages.

Ketamine can be given alone or in combination with xylazine or medetomidine. The latter combination has the advantage that anaesthesia can be reversed using atipamezole. The combinations can be given separately, or mixed in the same syringe, and given by intraperitoneal injection.

Ketamine/xylazine

Ketaset (Willows Francis Ltd.)

This contains 100 mg/ml ketamine.

Rompun (Bayer plc)

This contains 20 mg/ml xylazine.

Dose: 90 mg/kg ketamine plus 10 mg/kg xylazine can be given by intraperitoneal by injection.

Ketamine/medetomidine

Ketaset (Willows Francis Ltd.)

This contains 100 mg/ml ketamine.

Domitor (Pfizer Ltd.)

This contains 1 mg/ml medetomidine.

Dose: Ketamine 90 mg/kg plus 0.5 mg/kg medetomidine can be given by intraperitoneal injection.

Comment: This combination can be reversed with atipamezole (Anti-sedan, Pfizer Ltd.) at a dose of 1 mg/kg given by either subcutaneous or intraperitoneal injection.

Ketamine

Ketamine can be given alone for sedation at a dose rate of 22 mg/kg by intramuscular injection.

ANALGESIA

Buprenorphine

Vetergesic (Animalcare Ltd.)

This contains 0.3 mg/ml buprenorphine.

Dose: 0.05 mg/kg by subcutaneous injection every 8–12 hours. An average 500 g rat can be given 0.08 ml of Vetergesic.

Paracetamol

Rats find the paediatric suspensions quite palatable.

Calpol (Wellcome Ltd.)

The six plus suspension of Calpol contains 50 mg/ml paracetamol.

Dose: 100–300 mg/kg every 4 hours; a 500 g rat could be given 1.0 ml by mouth every 4 hours.

POST-OPERATIVE CARE

After anaesthesia a respiratory stimulant can be given. Doxapram (Dopram V, Willows Francis Ltd.) contains 20 mg/ml doxapram and can be given at a dose of 10–15 mg/kg by subcutaneous or intramuscular injection. Oxygen can also be administered via the face mask. Warmth is important; a light bulb makes a useful heat source.

Fluid replacement

Fluid replacement is important post-surgery, and at any other time when dehydration is a symptom. The fluid of choice is glucose/saline (0.9% NaCl, 5% glucose) and this should be warmed to body temperatured before being given by subcutaneous injection. The quantity for a rat is 16–32 ml. No more than 5 ml should be given at any one site.

INJECTION PROCEDURES

Subcutaneous injections can be made in the scruff of the neck, and up to 5 ml can be given by this route.

Intramuscular injections can be given into the quadriceps using a 23 gauge needle. The maximum volume that can be given in this site is 0.2 ml.

Intraperitoneal injections can be made with a 25 gauge needle. The rat should be held on its back with one hind leg extended. The needle can be introduced along the line of this leg into the centre of the corresponding posterior quadrant of the abdomen; 5 ml of fluid can be given by this route.

Intravenous injections are very difficult because of the small size of the patient; the lateral tail vein is used for this procedure.

DRUG TREATMENTS

Antibiotics

Tx 1. Enrofloxacin

Baytril (Bayer plc)

Dose: 10 mg/kg daily.

The 2.5% injection solution can be given subcutaneously at a dose of 0.2 ml/day. The 2.5% oral solution can be diluted 1:1 with blackcurrant syrup and given from a dropper bottle at a dose of 4 drops twice daily.

Drinking water can be medicated with the 2.5% oral solution to produce a concentration of 100 mg/litre by taking 4 ml and making it up to 1 litre with water.

Tx 2. Chloramphenicol

Chloramphenicol Injectable Suspension (Willows Francis Ltd.)

This contains 150 mg/ml chloramphenicol.

Dose: 10 mg/kg given by intramuscular injection twice daily. Chloramphenicol can also be given orally in the drinking water at a dose of 0.25 mg/ml. This concentration can be achieved by taking 1.7 ml of injectable suspension and making it up to 1 litre with water.

Tx 3. Neomycin

Neobiotic Aquadrops (Upjohn Ltd.)

These contain 50 mg/ml neomycin sulphate in a preservative.

Dose: The drinking water can be medicated at a rate of 2 g/litre. This concentration can be achieved by diluting 1 ml Aquadrops with 24 ml water.

Tx 4. Potentiated sulphonamides

Borgal 7.5% (Hoechst UK Ltd.)

This injection contains 62.5 mg/ml sulfadoxine and 12.5 mg/ml trimethoprim.

Dose: 1.5 ml/kg by subcutaneous injection. An average 500 g rat should receive 0.75 ml.

Tribrissen 24% (Mallinckrodt Veterinary Ltd.)

This injectable form contains 40 mg/ml trimethoprim and 200 mg/ml sulphadiazine.

Dose: It can be given orally in the drinking water at a dilution of 1:500, i.e. 1 ml made up to 0.5 litre with drinking water.

Tx 5. Sulphadimidine

Intradine (Norbrook Labs Ltd.)

This contains Sulphadimidine 33% w/v.

Dose: The required concentration in the drinking water is 0.2%. This dilution is achieved by taking 6 ml of Intradine and making it up to 1 litre with water.

Tx 6. Oxytetracycline

This antibiotic comes in various presentations, including a powder that can be mixed with water to make an oral solution, and short- and long-acting injectable preparations.

Terramycin LA Injectable (Pfizer Ltd.)

This is a long acting injection containing 200 mg/ml oxytetracycline.

Dose: 60 mg/kg by subcutaneous or intramuscular injection every 3 days. For an average 500 g rat this approximates to a dose of 0.15 ml.

Engemycin 5% (Mycofarm Ltd.)

This is a short acting injection containing 50 mg/ml oxytetracycline.

Dose: 100 mg/kg by subcutaneous injection daily. A dose for an average 500 g rat is 1 ml.

Terramycin Soluble Powder 5.5% (Pfizer Ltd.)

One level scoopful (about 4 g) of powder contains approximately 200 mg oxytetracycline.

Dose: The required concentration is 3 mg/ml. One level scoopful can be dissolved in 66 ml water to achieve this concentration.

Tx 7. Tylosin

Tylan 5. (Elanco Products Ltd.)

Each tablet contains 50 mg/ml tylosin.

Dose: 10 mg/kg may be given daily by subcutaneous injection.

Miscellaneous treatments

Tx 8. Corticosteroids

Betsolan injection (Mallinckrodt Veterinary Ltd.)

This contains 2 mg/ml betamethasone.

Dose: 0.1 mg/kg by subcutaneous injection. For an average 500 g rat this approximates to 0.025 ml.

Tx 9. Griseofulvin

Grisovin (Mallinckrodt Veterinary Ltd.)

This is an antifungal treatment, for the treatment of ringworm. Each Grisovin tablet contains 125 mg of griseofulvin.

Dose: Treatment should be continued for at least a month, at a dose of 25 mg/kg orally. An adult rat should be given one tenth of a tablet daily, crushed on the food.

Tx 10. Enilconazole

Imaverol (Jansen Animal Health)

This contains 100 mg/ml enilconazole.

Dose: Imaverol can be diluted 1:50 to provide a 0.2% w/v solution of enilconazole which can be used as a dip.

Tx 11. Ivermectin

Ivomec Injection for Cattle (Merck, Sharpe and Dohme)

This is an anti-parasitic injection containing 1% w/v ivermectin.

Dose: 200 µg/kg. Ivomec can be diluted 1:10, and a dose of 0.1 ml given by subcutaneous injection.

Alternatively Ivomec can be given orally at a dose of 1 drop by mouth (undiluted).

Treatment should be repeated after 10 days.

Tx 12. Amitraz

Aludex (Hoechst UK Ltd.)

This contains 50 g/l amitraz.

Dose: The recommended concentration is 0.01% (100 ppm) amitraz. This is achieved by diluting 1 ml Aludex in 0.5 litre of water. The solution should be used as a dip and not rinsed.

Tx 13. Kaolin/pectin

Kaogel (Parke Davis & Co Ltd.)

This contains 20% w/v light kaolin, and 0.43% w/v pectin.

Dose: 0.5 ml orally three times daily, as an adjunct to other diarrhoea therapy.

Comment: Many paediatric diarrhoea preparations are similar, and make suitable alternatives.

Tx 14. Metronidazole

This is an antibiotic with anti-protozoal activity.

Torgyl Solution (Rhône Mérieux Ltd.)

This contains 5 mg/ml metronidazole and can be diluted 1:1 with drinking water to provide a concentration of 2.5 mg/ml.

Flagyl-s Solution (Rhone Mérieux Ltd.)

This contains 40 mg/ml metronidazole and can be diluted 1:16 with drinking water to produce a concentration of 2.5 mg/ml.

Tx 15. Niclosamide

This is an anti-parasitic drug effective against cestodes.

Troscan 100 (Bayer plc.)

These tablets contain 100 mg niclosamide, and one half of a tablet can be given to an adult rat, and the dose repeated after 7 days. This approximates to a dose of 100 mg/kg.

Tx 16. Piperazine

This is an anti-parasitic drug effective against roundworms.

Antepar Elixir (Wellcome)

Antepar contains 150 mg/ml piperazine and this will control nematodes (pinworms).

Dose: The required concentration of 3 mg/ml piperazine in the drinking water can be achieved by diluting the elixir 1:50 with water, and replacing the drinking water with this solution.

Tx 17. Dermisol

Dermisol (Smith Kline Beecham)

This contains propylene glycol, malic acid, benzoic acid and salicylic acid. It promotes healing by removing dead and necrotic tissue from affected areas and also has antibacterial properties.

Dose: Dermisol can be applied to affected areas two or three times daily until the condition resolves.

Tx 18. Chloromycetin Ophthalmic Ointment 1% (Parke, Davis & Co. Ltd.)

This contains chloramphenicol and can be applied twice daily, or more frequently if required.

Tx 19. Chloromycetin Hydrocortisone Ophthalmic Ointment (Parke Davis & Co. Ltd.)

This contains chloramphenicol with hydrocortisone as the steroid. It can be applied twice daily.

Tx 20. Aureomycin Ophthalmic Ointment (Cyanamid UK Ltd.)

This contains 1% chlortetracycline hydrochloride. It can be applied twice daily.

Tx 21. Neobiotic HC (Upjohn Ltd.)

This contains the antibiotic neomycin with hydrocortisone as the steroid. It is a ready flowing liquid and can be applied two or three times daily.

Tx 22. Maxitrol (Alcon Ltd.)

This contains an antibiotic (neomycin), steroid (dexamethasone), and an antifungal agent (polymixin B). It can be applied two or three times daily.

Tx 23. Pyrethrin

Anti-mite Spray for Birds (Johnson)

This contains 0.8% w/v pyrethrin and piperonyl.

Dose: A light spray may be given and repeated weekly if necessary.

ZOONOTIC ASPECTS

INTRODUCTION

There are many and varied diseases documented as potential zoonoses in the literature. This section covers those that may be encountered in association with rodents kept as pets, or by the hobbyist for breeding and exhibiting.

ALLERGIC RESPONSES TO RODENTS

This is an important aspect to consider if a person becomes ill whilst keeping rodents. Allergic responses to the animal's bedding (particularly if it is hay or shavings) may occur. People may also develop cutaneous or respiratory allergies to rodent (mice and rat) dander or their urinary proteins. Clinical signs include itching, skin redness, ocular or nasal discharge, sneezing, and even difficulty in breathing. A sensitivity to rat urinary proteins may cause severe pulmonary allergies, and this is compounded if rats are kept in poor sanitary conditions and the urine is allowed to build up.

These allergic symptoms may be reduced if a mask and gloves are worn when handling the animals and cleaning their cages. The bedding material could be changed to shredded paper. It may also help to use a room air-filtration system.

ZOONOTIC DISEASES

Despite the range of potential zoonoses, there are only a few that may be significant in general practice. People with a healthy immune system will have a resistance to most diseases; however, if people are immunocompromised through concurrent disease, if they are young, or if they are taking immunosuppressive drugs, the risks of contracting a zoonotic disease are higher.

Wild rats and mice carry several diseases which may not occur in pets, but should be considered if wild rodents have access to the pets, or are able to soil their food or bedding.

Potential zoonoses are presented below in alphabetical order.

Cryptosporidiosis

Species affected: Rats, mice and hamsters.

Cryptosporidia has been implicated as a cause of diarrhoea in people with reduced immunocompetence, and in children under the age of 5 years. Symptoms include a profuse watery diarrhoea, occasionally with blood, colicky pains and anorexia. In immunocompetant people the disease is self-limiting. The organism is carried by hamsters, rats and mice, and is usually asymptomatic. Care must be taken when young children handle their pets, particularly if the pet has diarrhoea.

Giardiasis

Species affected: Hamsters and chinchillas.

Giardia spp. are found as inhabitants in the small intestine and are thought to be non-pathogenic. However it is possible for them to infect man and they may cause disease if the immune system is compromised.

Hymenolepiasis

Species affected: Hamsters, gerbils, rats and mice.

Hymenolepis nana, the dwarf tapeworm, is pathogenic for man and can cause enteric disease. Its control is difficult because it has three life cycle variations, only two of which can be controlled. The direct life cycle where eggs are passed in the faeces and ingested by the next rodent host can be controlled by regular cleaning of the environment. The indirect life cycle where the eggs are passed through insect vectors can also be controlled by insect control. However, the third cycle (autoinfection) where the eggs develop inside the intestinal lumen of the original host is less easily con-trolled, although the use of the drug niclosamide will help.

Lymphocytic choriomenigitis (LCM)

Species affected: Hamsters, rats and mice.

As yet this has been recorded in the USA, but may become a problem in other areas if stock is imported. It is transmitted via biting, and by contact with faeces or urine. Clinical signs in people range from influenza-like symptoms of fever and headaches, to a skin rash, arthritis and rarely a fatal encephalomyelitis.

Leptospirosis (Weil's disease)

Species affected: Rats.

Leptospira icterohaemorrhagiae [*Leptospira interrogans*] is carried by wild rats, and spread via water contaminated by rat urine. If rats gain access to the pet rodents' environment, or contaminate their food with urine, the infection can enter the pet colony.

Infection is transmitted to humans via ocular or nasal secretions, either entering through abrasions, or in aerosol form. Clinical signs in humans are vague influenza-like symptoms or weight loss.

Rat-bite fever

This is rare, but is caused by the bacterium *Streptobacillus moniliformis*, which may enter a colony via infected wild rats. The organism is carried by asymptomatic rats in the nasopharynx, and will infect humans through a rat bite. Clinical signs are a fever, petechial haemorrhages, and poly-arthritis.

Ringworm

Species affected: Chinchillas, hamsters, gerbils, mice and rats.

This is the commonest zoonosis, and is spread because the fungal spores are transferred when the affected animal is handled, or when contaminated bedding is touched. The most frequently isolated dermatophyte is

Trichophyton mentagrophytes though *Microsporum* spp. are also zoonotic.

Lesions on the owner are usually found on the hands and arms; these are small pruritic papules which increase in size to form the classic ring. Children may be particularly affected. To prevent human infection, proven or suspected cases in rodents should be handled with gloves, and only for the administration of treatment. Contaminated bedding can be burned, and cages washed out with a tertiary amine such as Trigene.

Salmonellosis

Species affected: Mice, rats, gerbils, chipmunks and hamsters.

Salmonella spp. should be considered in any case of intractable diarrhoea. Rats and mice may carry the disease subclinically and shed the bacteria to others. Birds and wild rodents must be excluded from the environment because they are often carriers of the disease. Once salmonellosis is identified elimination of the organism is difficult, and the most practical approach is to cull the existing stock, to disinfect the environment and utensils, and to restock.

Sarcoptic mange

Species involved: Rats and mice

This is rare in these rodents, and although theoretically a zoonosis, transmission is very rare, because the mite is a burrowing one and not immediately accessible.

Yersiniosis

Infection is spread by wild birds and rodents and contaminated foodstuffs. As for salmonellosis, a policy of culling, disinfection and restocking is advised.

DISINFECTANTS

There are many and varied disinfectants available. Their action on different classes of organisms, their effect on cage surfaces, and on animals that may be kept nearby are now reviewed. When using any disinfectant the manufacturer's instructions must be followed.

Biguanides

These have activity against bacteria and fungi. They are a useful skin disinfectant (e.g. Savlon, Hibbiscrub). They are very safe and non-irritant.

Tertiary amines

These may be formulated in combination with biguanide (e.g. Genie, Trigene). They are some of the safest disinfectants; they are non-irritant, non-corrosive and effective against bacteria, viruses, mycoplasms, fungi and their spores.

Phenolic compounds

Clear phenolic disinfectants (e.g. Jeyes fluid) are active against bacteria, fungi and mycoplasms. They are corrosive to surfaces, irritant to use, and irritant to in-contact animals.

Synthetic phenols (e.g. Dettol) are active against fungi and some bacteria; they are less irritant and non-corrosive.

Hyperchlorites (bleach)

Hypochlorites (e.g. Dosmestos) are active against bacteria, viruses, mycoplama, fungi and their spores. They are, however, highly corrosive, and irritant to the operator and in-contact animals.

Iodine-based compounds

These include Pevidine and Vanodine. The latter is non-toxic and can be put through drinking water containers to prevent bacterial contamination. Iodine-based compounds are active against bacteria, viruses and fungi. They are non-irritant.

Quaternary ammonium compounds

These are mainly bactericidal in action (e.g. Cetavlon). They are non-corrosive, but may be slightly irritant.

PHYSIOLOGICAL DATA

Chinchillas

Life span: 10 years
Adult weight: 400–500 g
Heart rate: 100–150/minute
Respiratory rate: 40–80/minute
Body temperature: 38°C (100°F)

Chipmunks

Life span: female, up to 8 years, average 4 years
        male, $2\frac{1}{2}$–5 years
Adult weight: 70–120 g
Respiration rate: 75/minute
Body temperature: 38°C (100°F), drops to environmental temperature during
  hibernation

Gerbils

Life span: 2–3 years
Adult weight: males 117 g
        females 100 g
Heart rate: 200–360/minute
Respiratory rate: 90–140/minute
Body temperature: 38°C (100°F)
Total blood volume (adult): 7 ml

Hamsters

Life span: Golden hamster 2 years
       Chinese hamster 2 years
       Russian hamster 9–15 months
Adult weight: golden male 85–130 g
       golden female 95–150 g
Heart rate: 300–600 (average 450)/minute
Respiration rate: 75/minute

Body temperature: 36–37.4°C (97–99°F)
Blood volume (adult): golden hamster 7 ml

Mice

Life span: 2–3 years
Adult weight: 20–40 g
Heart rate: 500–600/minute
Respiration rate: 100–250/minute
Body temperature: 37.5°C (99.5°F)
Blood volume (adult): 2.4–3 ml

Rats

Life span: 3–4 years
Adult weight: 400–800 g
Heart rate: 300–450/minute
Respiration rate: 70–150/minute
Body temperature: 38°C
Total blood volume (adult): 25–35 ml

REFERENCES

Chinchillas

Harris, J. (1987). *A Complete Guide to Chinchillas.* TFH Publications, USA.

Houston, J. and Prestwich, J. (1953). *Chinchilla Care.* Allied Fur Industries, California.

Kennedy, A.H. (1952). *Chinchilla Diseases and Ailments.* Clay Publishing Co., Bewdley.

Laber-Laird, K., Swindle, M. and Flecknell, P. (1996). *Handbook of Rodent and Rabbit Medicine.* Pergamon Press, Oxford.

Sweeney, A. (1996). *Extracts from Fur and Feather,* Printing for Pleasure, Ipswich.

Webb, R.A. (1991). *Chinchillas. Manual of Exotic Pets.* BSAVA, Cheltenham. pp. 19–23.

Chipmunks

Gillet, K. and Temple, J. (1991). *Chipmunks. Manual of Exotic Pets.* BSAVA, Cheltenham. pp. 23–30.

Henwood, C. (1989). *Chipmunks.* TFH Publications, USA.

Gerbils

Barrie, A. (1992). *The Proper Care of Gerbils.* TFH Publications, USA.

Flecknell, P. (1991). *Anaesthetic and Post-Operative Care of Small Mammals.* British Veterinary Association.

Harkness, J.E. and Wagner, J.E. (1989). *The Biology of Rabbits and Rodents.* Lea and Febiger, Philadelphia.

Toy, J. (1985). Gerbils. *Manual of Exotic Pets.* BSAVA, Cheltenham. pp. 28–35.

Laber-Laird, K., Swindle, M. and Flecknell, P. (1996). *Rodent and Rabbit Medicine.* Pergamon Press, Oxford.

McKellar, Q.A. (1989). *Drug Dosages for Small Mammals.* British Veterinary Association.

Hamsters

British Hamster Association Information Sheets. P.O. Box 825, Sheffield, England.

Flecknell, P. (1991). *Anaesthesia and Post-operative Care of Small Mammals.* In Practice. British Veterinary Association, London.

Harkness, J.E. and Wagner, J.E. (1989). *The Biology and Medicine of Rabbits and Rodents.* Lea and Febiger, Philadelphia.

Laber-Laird, K., Swindle, M. and Flecknell, P. (1996). *Rodent and Rabbit Medicine.* Pergamon Press, Oxford.

Mays, N. and Mays, M. (1991) *The Syrian Hamster.* Veterinary Practice.

McKay, J. (1991). *The New Hamster Handbook.* Strand, London.

Milward, P. (1996). *Extracts from Fur and Feather,* Printing for Pleasure, Ipswich.

Robinson. R. (1994). *The Right Way To Keep Hamsters.* Elliot Books, Surrey.

Toy, J. (1985). Hamsters. *Manual of Exotic Pets.* BSAVA, Cheltenham. pp. 45–53.

Mice

Bielfeld, H. (1984). *Mice, a Complete Pet Owner's Manual.* Barron's Educational Series.

Cook, A. (1977). *Exhibition and Pet Mice.* Spur Publications.

Flecknell, P. (1991). Rats and Mice. *Manual of Exotic Pets.* BSAVA, pp. 83–95. Cheltenham.

Harkness, J.E. and Wagner, J.E. (1989). *The Biology and Medicine of Rabbits and Rodents.* Lea and Febiger, Philadelphia.

Laber-Laird, K., Swindle, M. and Flecknell, P. (1996). *Rodent and Rabbit Medicine.* Pergamon, Oxford.

Malley, D. (1995). *Course Notes for BSAVA Continuing Education Course in Small Companion Animals.* BSAVA, Cheltenham.

McKellar, Q.A. (1989). *Drug Dosages for Small Mammals* In Practice. British Veterinary Association, London.

The Merck Veterinary Manual (1979). Merck and Co. Inc., New Jersey, USA.

Rats

Flecknell, P. (1991). Rats and Mice. *Manual of Exotic Pets.* BSAVA, pp. 83–95. Cheltenham.

Harkness, J.E. and Wagner, J.E. (1989). *The Biology and Medicine of Rabbits and Rodents.* Lea and Rebiger, Philadelphia.

Himsel, C.A. (1991). *Rats.* Barron's Educational Series.

Laber-Laird, K., Swindle, M. and Flecknell, P. (1995). *Rodent and Rabbit Medicine.* Pergamon, Oxford.

Malley, D. (1995). *Course notes for BSAVA Continuing Education course in Small Companion Animals.* BSAVA, Cheltenham.

Storey, A. (1996). *Extracts from Fur and Feather.* Printing for Pleasure, Ipswich.

INDEX